ISBN: 978-0-9941565-1-8

Layout and Design by Yvette Lillian Design Co

10 Secrets to Women's Radiant Health in Ayurveda

YVETTE LILLIAN

TIMELESS AYURVEDIC PRACTICES FOR
VIBRANT HEALTH AND INNER HARMONY

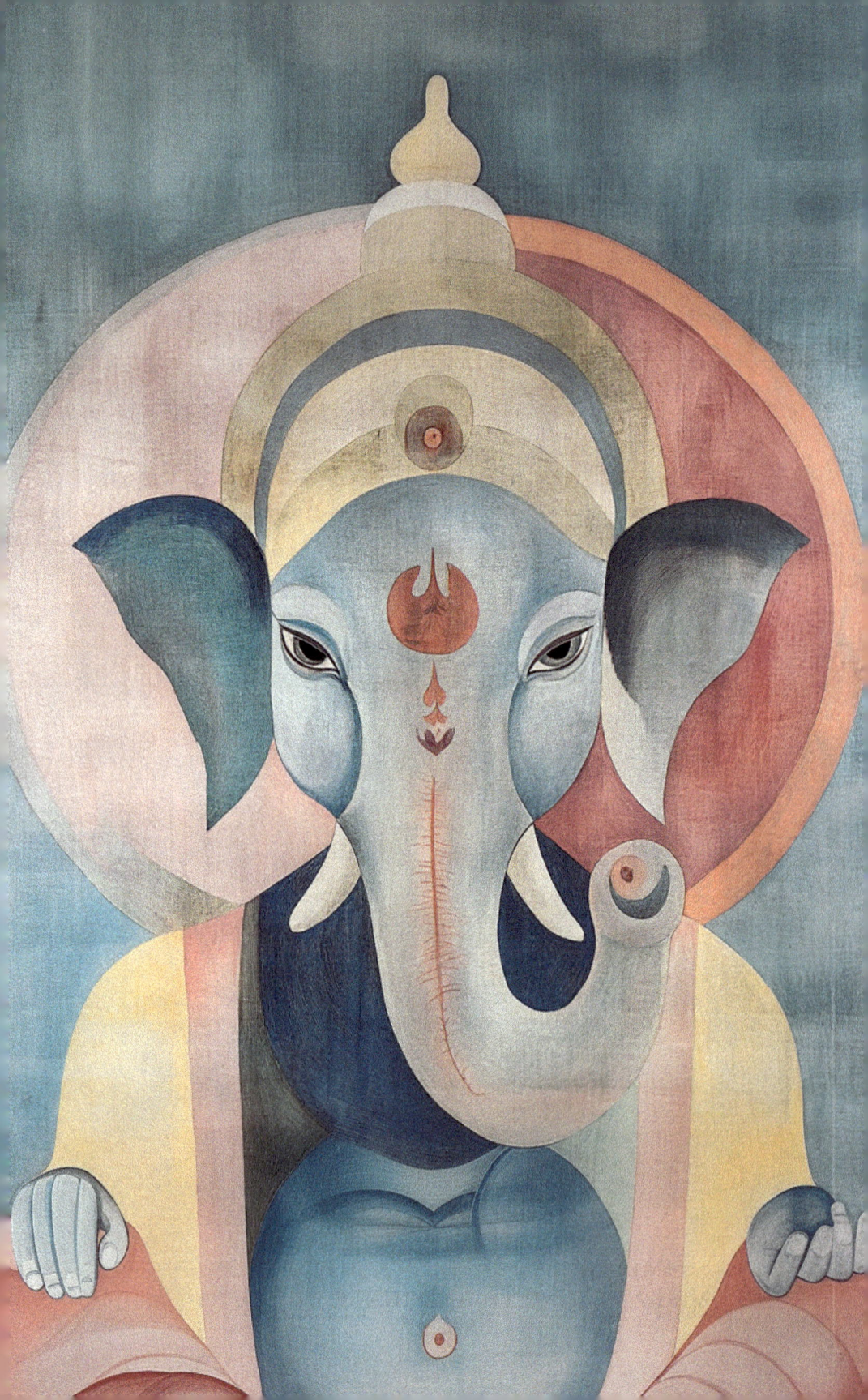

Contents

Introduction   01

Chapter 1: Understanding Ayurveda   05

Chapter 2: The Doshas   13

Secret 1: Discover Your Dosha   19

Chapter 3: Ayurvedic Nutrition   25

    Secret 2: You Are What You Digest   27

Chapter 4: Internal Cleansing   35

    Secret 3: Inner Detox for Outer Radiance   37

    Secret 4: Drinking the Nectar   38

    Secret 5: Body Exfoliation   40

    Secret 6: Oil Treatment   41

Chapter 5: Spiritual Harmony   45

    Secret 7: Exploring the Subtle Bodies   47

    Secret 8: Pranayama   49

    Secret 9: Find Your Joy   51

Chapter 6: Essential Oils for Ayurvedic Beauty   53

    Secret 10: The Right Skincare for You   55

Conclusion   61

Introduction

THE WORLD OF AYURVEDIC BEAUTY

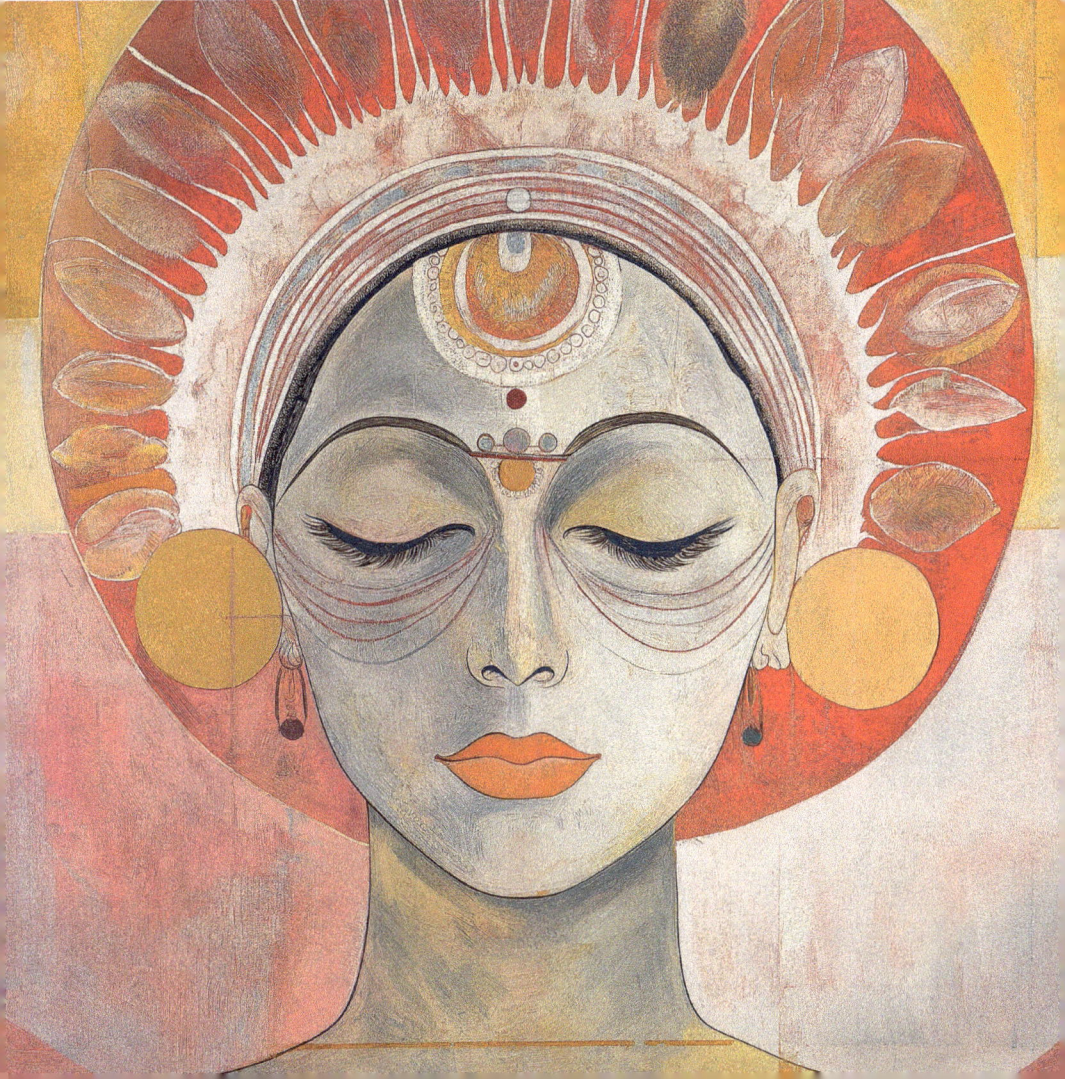

In Ancient Roots, Real Beauty Lives,
Not In What The Mirror Gives.
Ayurveda's Touch, Soft Yet True,
Brings Out The Light That's Deep In You.

Introduction
Welcome to the Transformative World of Ayurvedic Beauty

Welcome to the transformative world of Ayurvedic beauty—a timeless approach that celebrates your natural radiance, moving beyond the fleeting standards often showcased in glossy magazine spreads. Rooted in ancient wisdom, Ayurveda nurtures beauty from within, fostering a harmonious balance between body, mind, and spirit that transcends mere surface appearances.

In today's fast-paced society, the pressure to conform to societal beauty ideals can often leave women feeling disconnected from their true selves. Ayurveda, an age-old system of holistic health, offers a refreshing alternative by viewing beauty not as something applied externally, but as a genuine reflection of inner balance and well-being.

Known as the "science of life," Ayurveda's enduring principles of balance, nourishment, and self-care have withstood the test of time. These teachings are especially empowering for women seeking to reclaim their vitality and natural glow amidst the demands of modern living. Unlike transient beauty trends, Ayurveda emphasizes nurturing both body and mind, enhancing your innate beauty from the inside out.

Embracing this approach is not merely a luxury—it's a vital practice for navigating the stresses and challenges of today's world.

This book invites you on a heartfelt journey of self-discovery and empowerment. You will uncover your unique constitution and learn how to cultivate beauty that is authentic, lasting, and deeply connected to your overall well-being. Through Ayurveda's ten timeless secrets, you'll gain the knowledge and tools to nurture yourself holistically, achieving a luminous glow that signifies physical health, mental clarity, and spiritual harmony—a beauty that is sustainable, meaningful, and uniquely yours.

This journey into Ayurvedic beauty is more than an external makeover; it's an opportunity to reconnect with your essence. Ayurveda honours the true beauty within every woman, guiding you towards self-care practices that align with your individuality and radiance. Here, beauty is not a goal to chase but a natural state that emerges from balance, health, and mindful living. As you explore these practices, you'll find that true beauty feels as good as it looks, revealing itself as an enduring harmony of body, mind, and spirit. Embrace this journey as a way to feel profoundly connected to yourself and the world around you, nurturing a beauty that grows from within.

Chapter 1

UNDERSTANDING AYURVEDA

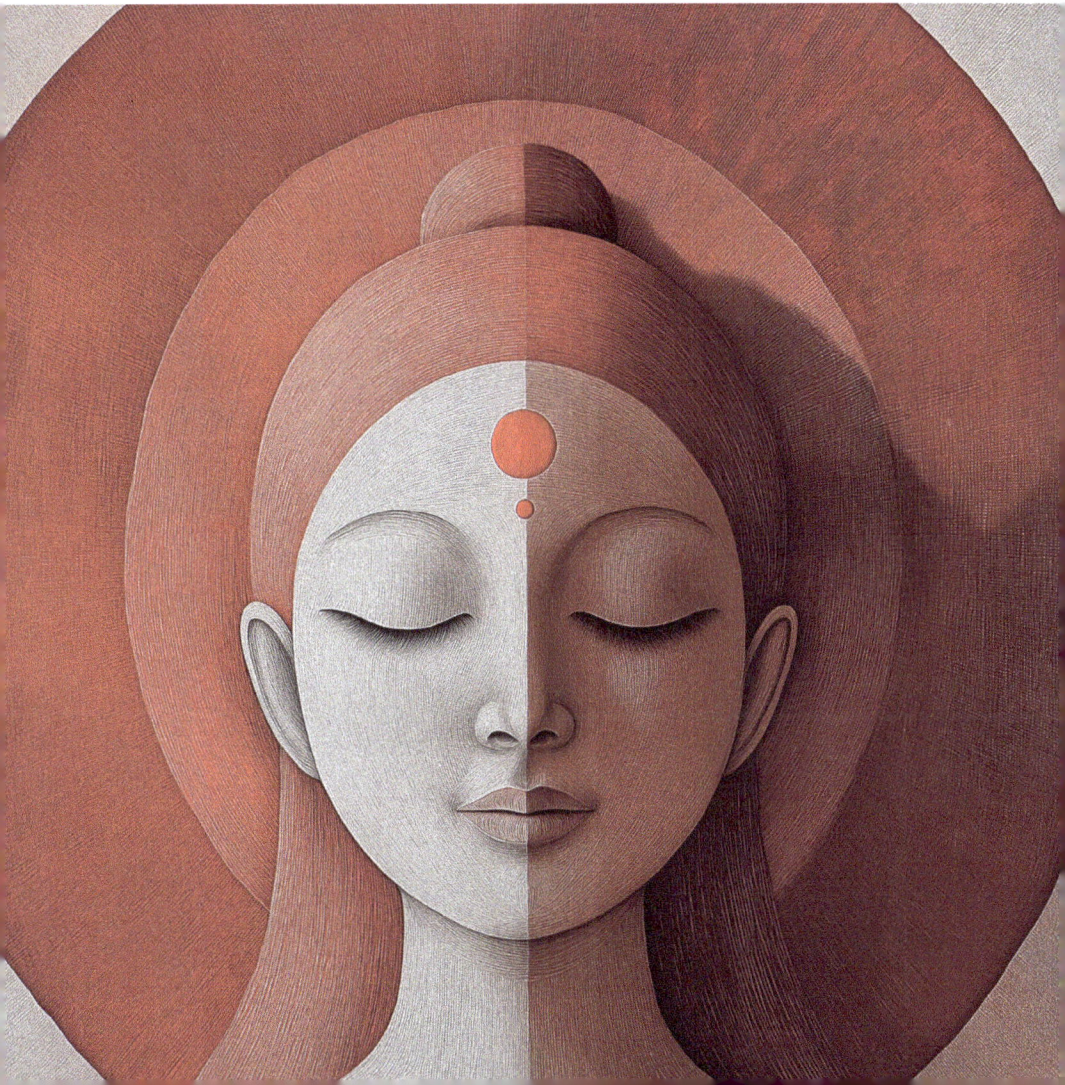

A Beauty That Whispers From Balance And Peace,
In Ayurveda's Wisdom, All Worries Cease.
Harmony Unfolds, As Body And Soul Entwine,
Revealing A Glow That's Uniquely Divine.

Chapter 1:
Understanding Ayurveda
The Ancient Art of Holistic Healing

Ayurveda, meaning "science of life" in Sanskrit, is a profound system of health and wellness developed over 5,000 years ago in India. Known as the "Mother of All Healing," Ayurveda's insights into the natural world and human body laid the foundation for many traditional and modern health systems. This ancient practice goes beyond treating symptoms to address the root cause of illness, recognising the body as a deeply interconnected system. Ayurveda's core goal is to maintain a balanced state of health and wellness through harmony within the body, mind, and spirit—a philosophy that is increasingly relevant today.

The Origins and Sacred Texts of Ayurveda

Ayurveda's roots are embedded in Indian culture and spirituality. Originally passed down orally by sages who studied the rhythms of nature and the human body, Ayurveda's wisdom was eventually preserved in sacred texts such as the **Caraka Samhita, Sushruta Samhita, and Astanga Hridaya.** These revered texts continue to be the foundation of Ayurvedic knowledge, encompassing a vast range of topics, including anatomy, diet, lifestyle, mental health, and spiritual practices.

Each Text Offers Unique Insights Into Ayurvedic Philosophy:

- **The Caraka Samhita** explores disease prevention and treatment, offering detailed guidance on lifestyle, diet, and the mental aspects of health.
- **The Sushruta Samhita** introduces foundational concepts of surgery, anatomy, and pathology, revealing an advanced understanding of medicine.
- **The Astanga Hridaya**, a combination of the previous texts, presents a complete guide to Ayurveda with a focus on both prevention and rejuvenation practices.

Ayurveda is a science rooted in respect for nature, viewing the human body as a microcosm of the greater universe (macrocosm). This philosophy of interconnectedness shapes Ayurveda's approach to wellness: rather than isolating symptoms, it considers each person's unique physical, mental, and spiritual attributes.

The Ayurvedic Perspective on Health and Wellness

Ayurveda teaches that true wellness is achieved when we create balance within ourselves and in our relationship with the world around us. It recognises that each individual is a unique blend of energies and that health is a dynamic state that requires continuous adaptation and awareness. In Ayurveda, well-being is not only defined by physical health but by a harmonious state of body, mind, and spirit.

The Five Elements

According to Ayurveda, everything in the universe, including the human body, is composed of five fundamental elements: **Earth, Water, Fire, Air, and Ether (Space)**. Each element represents a unique quality:

- **Earth:** Stability, structure, and solidity, representing our bones, muscles, and tissues.
- **Water:** Fluidity, cohesion, and flow, symbolising blood, lymph, and bodily fluids.
- **Fire:** Transformation, digestion, and metabolism, present in our ability to process food, thoughts, and emotions.
- **Air:** Movement, lightness, and adaptability, governing bodily functions such as breathing and circulation.
- **Ether:** (Space): Expansion, freedom, and openness, the basis of consciousness and the mind's capacity for awareness.

In Ayurveda, the three doshas—**Vata, Pitta, and Kapha**—govern physical and mental processes. Each person's unique constitution, or **Prakruti**, blends these doshas and stays fairly constant. However, factors like lifestyle, seasons, and environment can disrupt this balance, creating a temporary state called **Vikruti**. Ayurveda helps us recognise these shifts and restore harmony.

The Three Doshas: Vata, Pitta, and Kapha

Each of the three doshas embodies specific qualities and governs various physiological and psychological processes in the body.

Vata Dosha: Composed of Air and Ether, Vata is the energy of movement and governs all motion in the body, from blood circulation to cellular activity. When in balance, Vata promotes creativity, adaptability, and enthusiasm. When out of balance, it can cause anxiety, dryness, digestive issues, and restlessness. Vata is often associated with dry, thin skin, a lean frame, and irregular digestion. People with a Vata constitution are typically energetic and expressive, though they may be prone to stress and worry when Vata becomes excessive.

Pitta Dosha: Composed of Fire and Water, Pitta is the energy of transformation and governs digestion, metabolism, and body temperature. Balanced Pitta manifests as intelligence, courage, and determination. When unbalanced, it can lead to anger, irritability, and inflammation. Pitta types often have warm, oily skin, a medium build, and a strong appetite. They are ambitious, focused, and driven, with sharp mental clarity, but may experience irritability, skin rashes, or digestive issues when Pitta is out of balance.

Kapha Dosha: Made of Earth and Water, Kapha is the energy of stability, structure, and lubrication, governing immunity and the body's structural integrity. When in balance, Kapha embodies compassion, patience, and resilience. When out of balance, it can lead to lethargy, weight gain, and attachment. Kapha types usually have smooth, radiant skin, sturdy frames, and strong immunity. They are calm and nurturing but may become resistant to change and struggle with sluggishness if Kapha becomes excessive.

Each person has a unique doshic makeup, with one or two doshas dominant. Understanding this helps us make choices to support balance and improve health.

The Three Pillars of Ayurvedic Health

To sustain balance within the body, Ayurveda emphasises three foundational pillars:

Balanced Doshas: The harmony between Vata, Pitta, and Kapha is essential for physical and mental wellness. By making choices aligned with our doshic needs, we can support a balanced internal environment, reducing the likelihood of illness.

Agni (Digestive Fire): Ayurveda considers digestion to be the cornerstone of health. A strong Agni transforms food into energy, thoughts into insight, and experiences into wisdom. Imbalanced Agni can lead to toxicity, sluggishness, and illness, which is why Ayurveda places great importance on mindful eating and foods that suit one's dosha.

A Healthy Mind (Manas): Ayurveda views the mind as equally important as the body, recognising that mental and emotional well-being significantly impact physical health. Practices such as meditation, self-reflection, and pranayama (breathing exercises) are encouraged to cultivate mental clarity, emotional resilience, and peace.

Ayurveda's Approach to Health in the Modern World

In today's fast-paced world, environmental toxins, stressful routines, processed foods, and constant digital engagement often disrupt our natural balance, leading to physical and mental strain. Ayurveda offers a pathway to reconnect with our inherent nature and restore this balance through practical, sustainable practices.

Dinacharya (Daily Routine): Ayurvedic routines help establish regularity and reduce stress by incorporating practices like oil pulling, abhyanga (self-massage), and meditation. These rituals support cleansing, relaxation, and overall vitality.

Ritucharya (Seasonal Adjustments): Ayurveda acknowledges that seasonal changes affect our bodies and recommends adjustments to diet, exercise, and self-care to remain balanced year-round. For example, light, cooling foods are suggested in summer, while warming, nourishing foods are beneficial in winter.

Mindful Eating: Ayurveda teaches that how we eat is as important as what we eat. Eating mindfully, according to our doshic needs, and with gratitude helps us digest more efficiently and maintain energy levels.

Stress Management and Self-Care: Ayurveda recognises the harmful effects of chronic stress and provides tools like meditation, yoga, and breathing exercises to cultivate calm and resilience. These practices not only support mental health but also prevent doshic imbalances and boost immunity.

Prakruti and Vikruti: Discovering Your Unique Constitution

In Ayurveda, knowing your Prakruti—your unique, natural constitution—is fundamental to achieving and maintaining health. Your Prakruti reflects the balance of the doshas that were present at the time of your conception, serving as your individual blueprint for wellness. However, factors like stress, environment, diet, and lifestyle can shift this balance, creating a temporary state called Vikruti, which represents your current doshic state.

Recognising your Vikruti allows you to understand how your current state may differ from your original constitution, helping you make adjustments to restore balance. Ayurveda empowers us with this knowledge, showing that health is a dynamic state that can be influenced and improved through conscious choices.

Ayurveda's Path to Inner and Outer Radiance

Ayurveda's approach to beauty and wellness goes beyond the surface, focusing on inner harmony that radiates outward. By balancing the doshas, supporting Agni, and nourishing the mind, it promotes natural, sustainable beauty. True wellness lies in embracing our unique qualities rather than external standards. Ayurveda teaches that beauty stems from inner balance, just as health arises from a harmonious lifestyle. By honouring our doshic constitution, aligning with nature, and practising self-care, we can lead vibrant, fulfilling, and radiant lives.

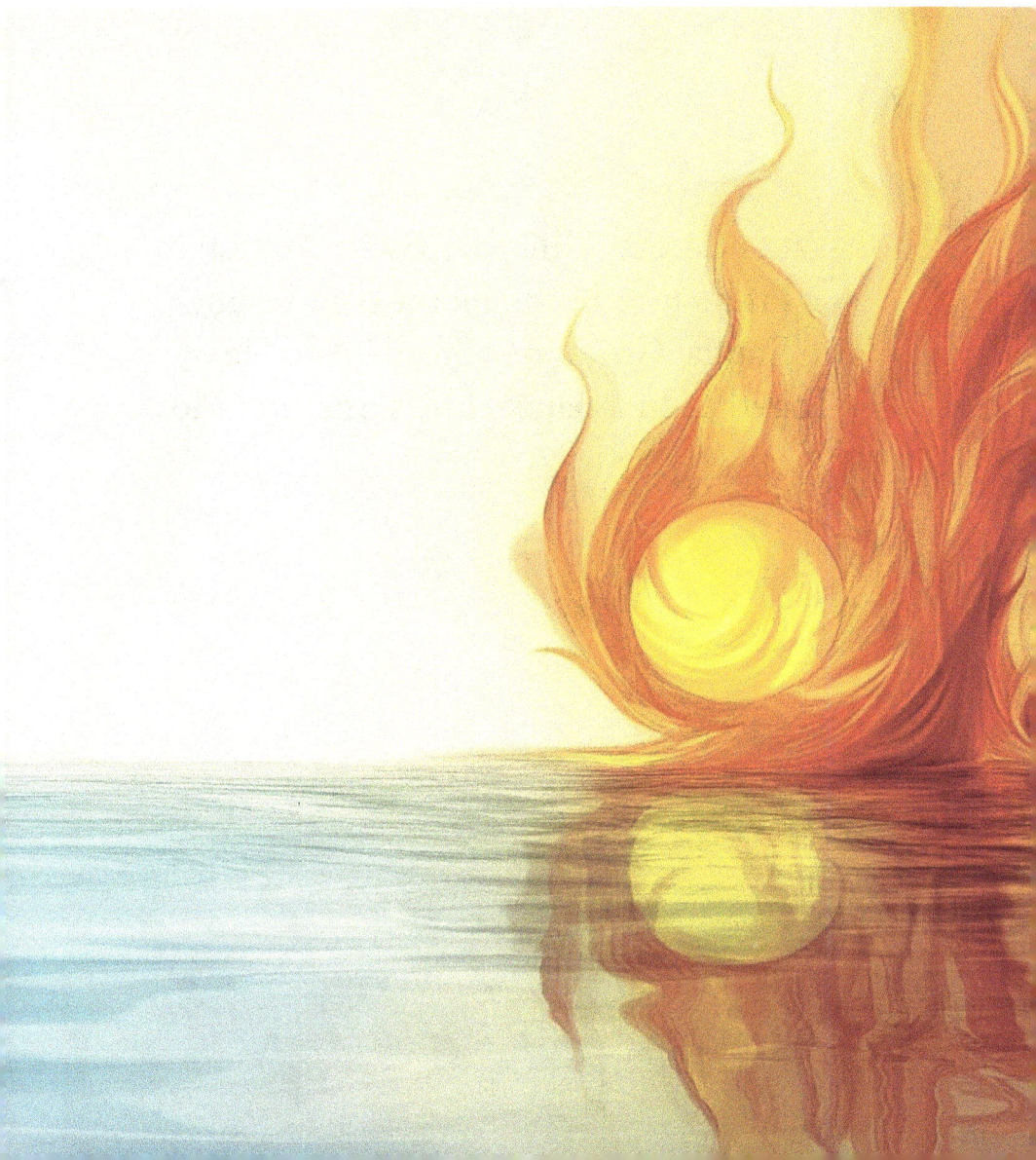

Chapter 2

THE DOSHAS

Vata's Breeze Whispers, Swift And Light,
Pitta's Fire Burns Fierce And Bright.
Kapha, Grounded, Steady And Slow,
Together In Balance, Life's Energies Flow

Chapter 2:
The Doshas
Unveiling the Essence Of Your Nature

At the heart of Ayurveda lies the concept of the doshas, which are the three primary energies that govern all physical, mental, and emotional processes in the body. These doshas—Vata, Pitta, and Kapha—are derived from the five elements (Earth, Water, Fire, Air, and Ether) and represent a unique blend of these elements. Together, the doshas shape our constitution, behaviour, tendencies, and even our preferences and vulnerabilities. Understanding the doshas provides insight into our natural state of balance and illuminates the path to optimal health and beauty.

In Ayurveda, each person has a Prakruti, or natural constitution, which is a distinct combination of the three doshas. While all three doshas are present in everyone, most people have one or two dominant doshas that define their physical, mental, and emotional characteristics. Recognising our doshic constitution is a key step in understanding how to make lifestyle, dietary, and self-care choices that align with our unique needs, thus restoring and maintaining balance.

The doshas also fluctuate in response to various factors such as diet, lifestyle, climate, and emotional states. This dynamic balance between the doshas is a natural process, but significant or prolonged imbalances can lead to discomfort, health issues, or a sense of being "out of alignment." Ayurveda empowers us to identify these imbalances and adopt practices that bring us back to our natural state of wellness.

Vata Dosha: The Energy of Movement and Change

Vata is the dosha composed of Air and Ether (Space), embodying the qualities of lightness, dryness, coldness, roughness, subtlety, and mobility. It governs all movement in the body, from breathing to muscle

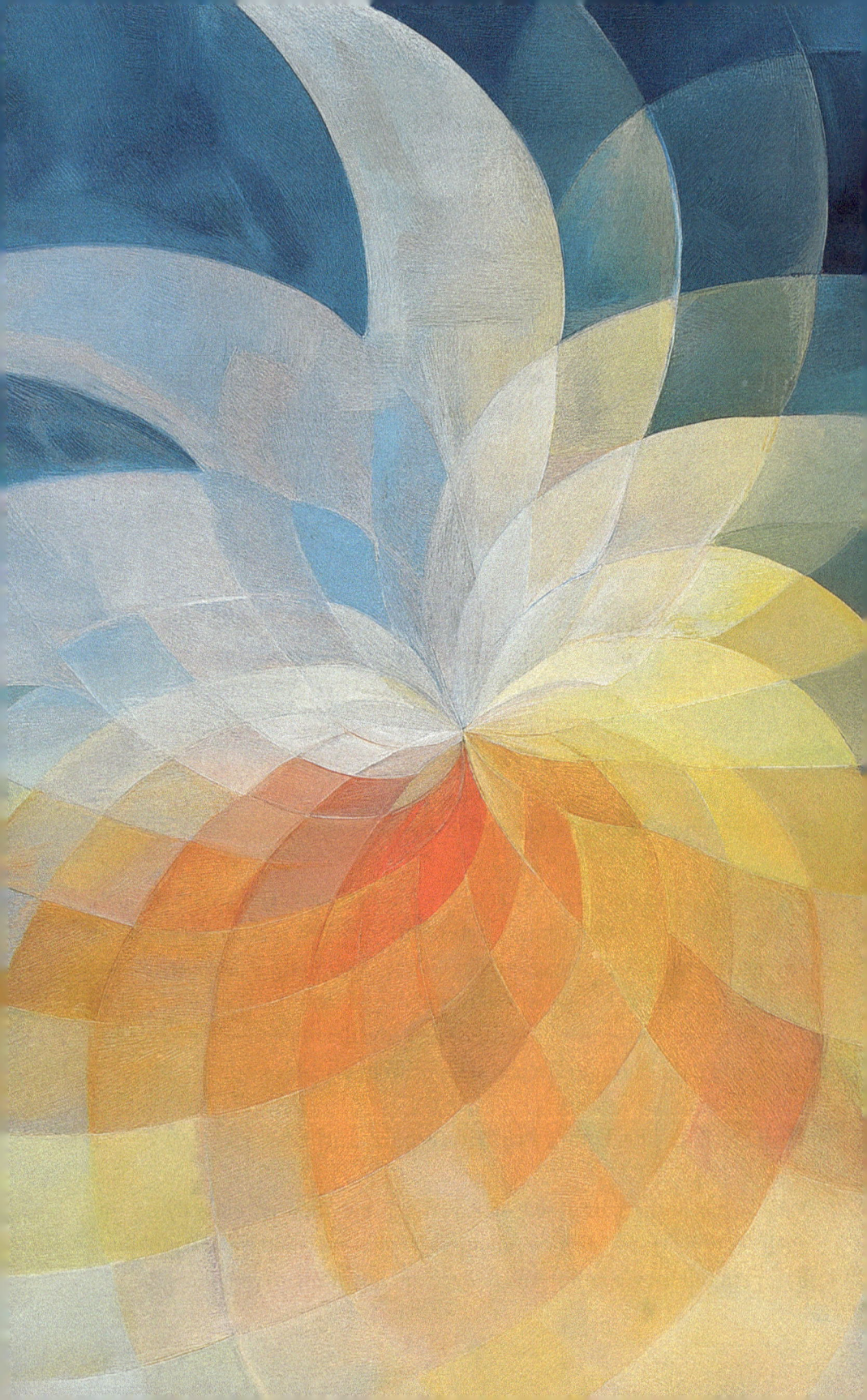

contractions, blood flow, and even the blinking of the eyes. Vata is often described as the "wind" within the body, responsible for our creative energy, flexibility, and adaptability.

People with a Vata-dominant constitution are typically energetic, expressive, and enthusiastic. They are naturally creative and often have a love for new experiences and travel. Physically, Vata types tend to have a slender frame, with dry skin, cold hands and feet, and prominent bone structure. They are quick thinkers, but when Vata is out of balance, it can lead to restlessness, anxiety, fear, digestive issues, and insomnia.

The influence of Vata is most pronounced during the autumn and early winter months, which are cool, dry, and windy. During this time, Vata types may feel the need for warmth, grounding, and regularity to counterbalance these qualities. Vata is also more likely to increase in times of stress, erratic schedules, or when we consume cold or raw foods. To bring Vata back into balance, Ayurveda recommends warm, nourishing foods, routine, and grounding practices that provide stability and warmth.

Pitta Dosha: The Energy of Transformation and Metabolism

Pitta is composed of Fire and Water, representing the qualities of heat, sharpness, lightness, intensity, and oiliness. Pitta governs the processes of digestion, absorption, and metabolism, as well as the mind's ability to process information and solve problems. Just as fire transforms fuel into heat, Pitta transforms food into energy and information into understanding.

Individuals with a Pitta-dominant constitution are often characterised by a medium, athletic build, warm skin tone, and a sharp mind. Pitta types are known for their focus, intelligence, and ambition, with a natural ability to organise and lead. However, when Pitta is aggravated, it can manifest as anger, irritability, inflammation, and sensitivity, particularly in the skin and digestive system. Balancing Pitta involves cooling activities, calming practices, and a diet rich in soothing, nourishing foods.

Pitta's influence is strongest during the summer months, which are hot and intense. In hot weather or when consuming spicy foods, Pitta types may feel overheated or irritable. Balancing Pitta involves cooling and soothing practices, such as spending time in nature, consuming cooling foods (like cucumbers and leafy greens), and avoiding intense heat and competitive situations.

Kapha Dosha: The Energy of Structure and Stability

Kapha is composed of Earth and Water and embodies the qualities of heaviness, steadiness, coldness, oiliness, smoothness, and solidity. Kapha provides structure and stability to the body, maintaining immunity, strength, and the lubrication of tissues. Kapha is often described as the "earth" within us, keeping us grounded, calm, and resilient.

Those with a Kapha-dominant constitution generally have a strong, solid build, smooth and radiant skin, and a calm, nurturing demeanour. Kapha types are naturally patient, compassionate, and supportive, known for their endurance and stability. When Kapha is out of balance, however, it can lead to lethargy, attachment, weight gain, and resistance to change.

Kapha's influence is most noticeable in the spring season, which is characterised by dampness and heaviness. During this time, Kapha types may feel an increased sense of sluggishness or congestion, which can be balanced through invigorating practices like regular exercise, lighter foods, and activities that bring variety and movement into their lives.

The Balance of the Doshas

While most people have one or two dominant doshas, everyone contains all three doshas to some degree. Ayurveda teaches that true wellness comes from a dynamic balance among these doshas. Our constitution, or Prakruti, is the natural balance we were born with, but daily choices, stressors, and environmental factors can shift this balance, creating an imbalance or Vikruti. By understanding our Prakruti and Vikruti, we can make lifestyle and dietary adjustments that support a return to balance.

Secret 1: Discover Your Dosha

Understanding your dosha is the first step in the Ayurvedic journey to holistic beauty and wellness. Each dosha shapes not only physical characteristics but also mental and emotional tendencies. By identifying your dosha, you gain insight into how your body, mind, and spirit respond to various influences, enabling you to make choices that enhance balance and harmony.

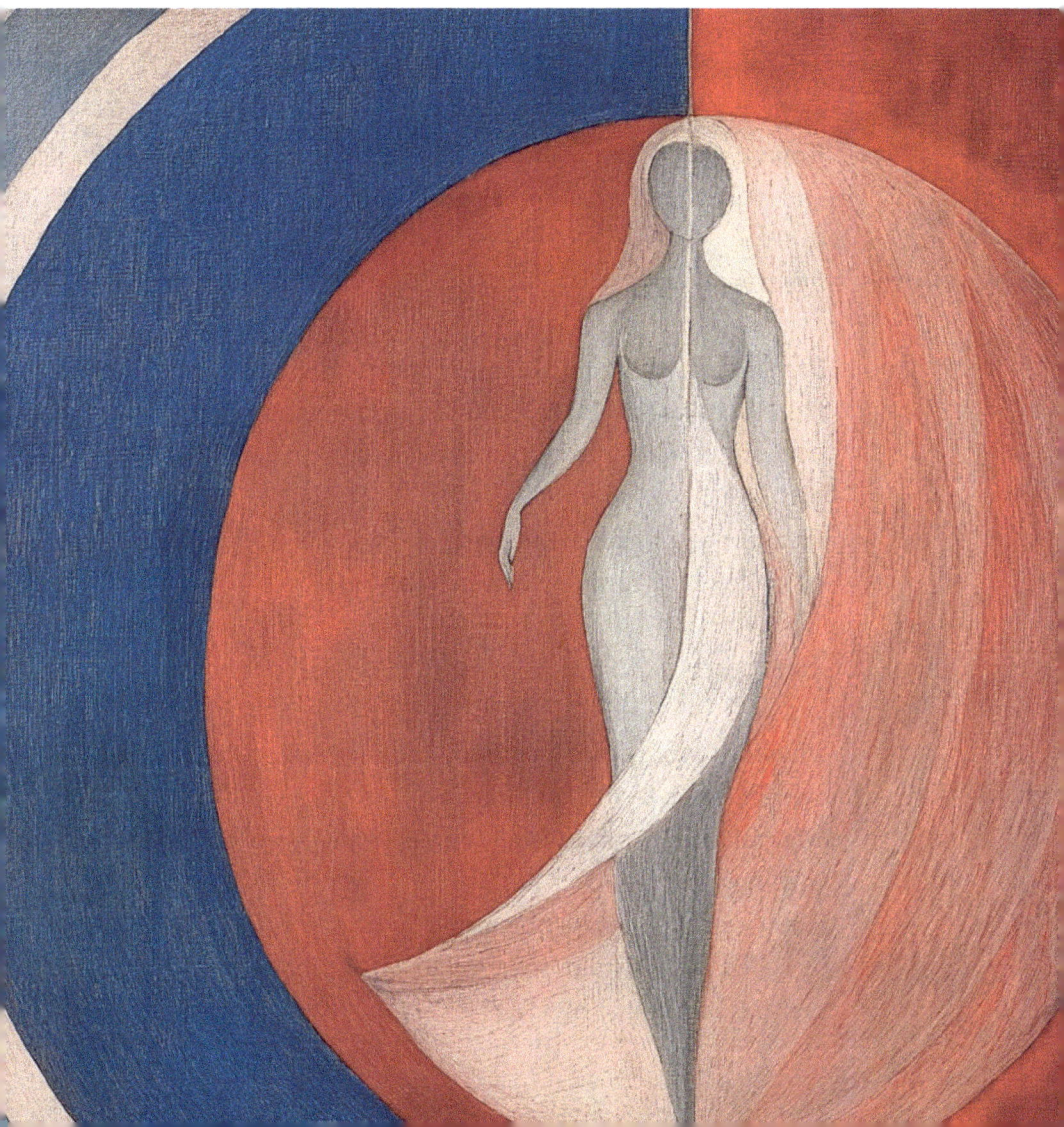

How to Discover Your Dosha

Discovering your dosha can be done through self-assessment and awareness of your body's tendencies, both physically and mentally. While an Ayurvedic practitioner can provide a detailed assessment, here are some basic characteristics associated with each dosha to help guide your exploration.

Vata Characteristics

- **Physical:** Thin, light frame; dry skin and hair; cold hands and feet; quick movement and speech.
- **Mental:** Creative, energetic, and adaptable but prone to anxiety and worry.
- **Emotional:** Sensitive and enthusiastic but can experience fear and restlessness when imbalanced.

Pitta Characteristics

- **Physical:** Medium build, warm body temperature, tendency to freckled or reddish skin, prone to inflammation.
- **Mental:** Intelligent, sharp, and focused, with a natural ability to plan and organise.
- **Emotional:** Passionate, driven, and confident, but can become irritable or aggressive when imbalanced.

Kapha Characteristics:

- **Physical:** Sturdy build, smooth and oily skin, tendency to gain weight easily, strong endurance.
- **Mental:** Calm, steady, and loyal, with excellent long-term memory.
- **Emotional:** Compassionate and loving, though may become attached or resistant to change when imbalanced, prone to feelings of melancholy.

Practical Tips for Balancing Your Dosha

Once you've identified your primary dosha, you can begin to incorporate practices that align with your constitution. Here are some practical tips for balancing each dosha:

Vata Balancing

- Embrace warmth and stability in diet, lifestyle, and environment.
- Eat warm, cooked foods with oils and spices to soothe dryness and coldness.
- Establish a regular daily routine with time for rest and reflection.
- Engage in grounding exercises like yoga and meditation.

Pitta Balancing

- Incorporate cooling, soothing foods like cucumbers, leafy greens, and coconut water.
- Avoid overly spicy, salty, or fried foods, which can aggravate Pitta.
- Spend time in nature, particularly near water, to soothe the mind and body.
- Practise moderation in work and exercise to prevent burnout and irritability.

Kapha Balancing

- Engage in regular physical activity, particularly invigorating exercise that stimulates circulation.
- Focus on light, warming foods with spices like ginger and black pepper.
- Limit heavy, oily, or sugary foods, which can increase Kapha's tendency for sluggishness.
- Incorporate variety and stimulation into your routine to keep energy levels up.

Your Doshas Reveals The Rhythm Within,
A Map To Your Balance, Where Health Can Begin.
Embrace Each Quality, Gentle And Kind,
A Guide To The Harmony Of Body And Mind.

Embracing Your Unique Constitution

Understanding your dosha is about embracing your unique constitution and learning how to work with it to create harmony within yourself. Ayurveda teaches that beauty and wellness are deeply personal, and that each person has a unique path to follow. Your dosha is not a label or limitation; rather, it is a guide to help you understand your strengths and areas where you may need support. By honouring and nurturing your constitution, you can achieve a sense of well-being that radiates from within, reflecting a balanced state of body, mind, and spirit.

The Benefits of Knowing Your Dosha

- **Empowers Health Choices:** By understanding your unique tendencies, you can make daily choices that support your health and well-being.
- **Personalised Self-Care:** Ayurveda offers dosha-specific guidance for everything from diet to exercise, skincare, and mental health practices.
- **Insight into Relationships:** Awareness of doshic qualities can enhance relationships by helping us understand others' natural tendencies and approach them with compassion.
- **A Path to Self-Acceptance:** Understanding your dosha encourages self-acceptance, helping you appreciate and work with your unique nature rather than resisting it.

By discovering and embracing your dosha, you begin a journey of self-understanding that is both empowering and transformative. Ayurveda provides a compassionate, holistic approach to wellness that honours individuality, guiding you to a balanced, radiant, and harmonious life. As you explore the ten secrets of Ayurvedic beauty in this book, remember that each principle is designed to help you deepen your understanding of yourself, creating a beauty that is authentic, sustainable, and deeply rewarding fulfilling. This journey is not just about outer beauty but also about cultivating inner peace and vitality.

Chapter 3

AYURVEDIC NUTRITION

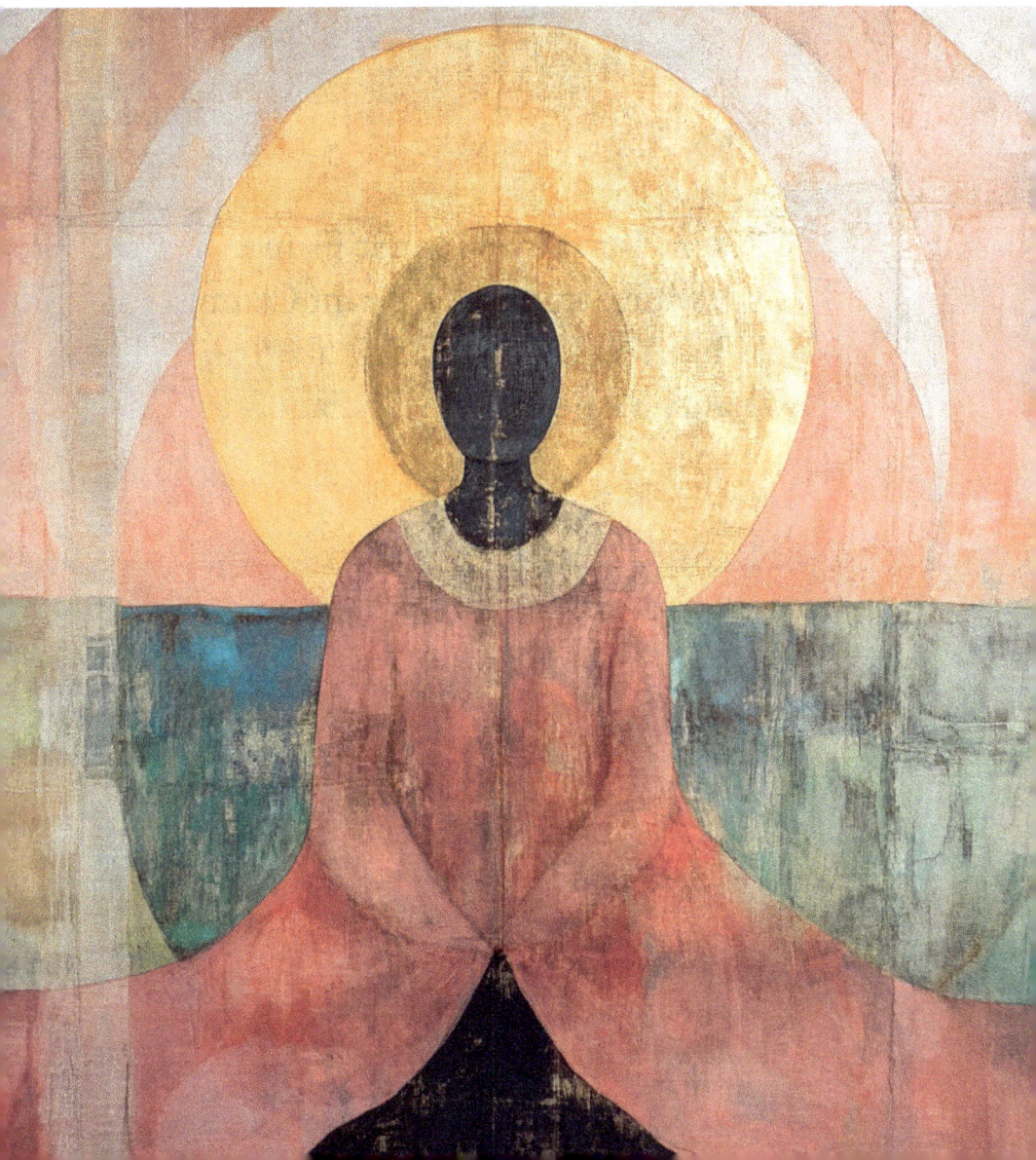

Agni Burns, The Inner Flame,
Digestion Strong, A Vibrant Claim.
What You Digest, You Truly Are,
Vitality Shines Like A Radiant Star.

Chapter 3:
Ayurvedic Nutrition
Embracing the Power of Digestion
Inner and Outer Radiance

In Ayurveda, digestion is considered the cornerstone of health, determining not only how well we absorb nutrients but also how clearly we think, how stable we feel emotionally, and how radiant we appear.

The Ayurvedic approach to nutrition goes far beyond counting calories or following dietary trends. Instead, it views food as a powerful tool for balancing our unique constitution and nurturing our vitality from within.

Central to Ayurveda's nutritional wisdom is the concept of Agni, or the digestive fire. Agni is responsible for transforming food into the energy that fuels every process in the body. When Agni is strong and balanced, we feel energised, mentally clear, and in harmony with ourselves. When Agni is weak, however, food is not properly digested, leading to the accumulation of toxins, known as Ama, which can manifest as dull skin, low energy, indigestion, and even mood disturbances.

This chapter explores how to nurture and strengthen Agni to ensure that food becomes a source of energy, clarity, and beauty rather than a contributor to imbalance. Secret 2, "**You Are What You Digest**," introduces the essential role of Agni in Ayurvedic nutrition and offers practical guidance on how to eat according to your dosha to optimise digestion and wellness.

The phrase "you are what you digest" captures the essence of Ayurveda's approach to food and nutrition. While modern dietary advice focuses on what to eat, Ayurveda places equal emphasis on how we digest and assimilate these foods. Agni, the digestive fire, transforms what we consume into tissues, energy, and mental clarity needed to thrive. A balanced Agni ensures we gain maximum benefit from food, while a weak or imbalanced Agni can lead to a buildup of toxins (Ama).

Understanding Agni – The Digestive Fire

In Ayurveda, Agni is viewed as a sacred force, the inner fire that fuels all physical and mental processes. Agni governs the digestion, absorption, assimilation, and transformation of food into energy. It also plays a critical role in mental clarity and emotional stability. When Agni is balanced, we experience good digestion, steady energy, mental focus, and vibrant health. When Agni is weak, however, undigested food turns into Ama, which clogs our systems and manifests as dull skin, lethargy, digestive discomfort, and even negative thought patterns.

Agni is affected by a variety of factors, including diet, lifestyle, emotional state, environment, and seasonal changes. For example, eating large meals late at night, consuming processed foods, or experiencing prolonged stress can all weaken Agni. On the other hand, eating with mindfulness, consuming dosha-appropriate foods, and maintaining a balanced lifestyle can strengthen Agni and support overall health.

A Balanced Agni Reflects Optimal Digestion:

- A feeling of lightness after meals
- Regular and comfortable bowel movements
- High energy levels throughout the day
- Clear and focused thinking
- Radiant skin and a healthy glow
- A strong immune system and resistance to illness

Signs Of Imbalanced Or Weak Agni Include:

- Bloating, gas, or constipation
- Feeling heavy or sluggish after meals
- Unusual cravings, particularly for processed or sugary foods
- Lethargy, low energy, and mental fog
- Skin issues such as breakouts or dullness
- Frequent colds, infections, or a weakened immune system

Types Of Agni And Their Influence On Digestion

In Ayurveda, Agni can fluctuate in various ways, and recognising your type of Agni can help you tailor your eating habits for balance:

Sama Agni (Balanced Agni): This type of Agni is stable and balanced, resulting in good digestion, assimilation, and elimination. People with Sama Agni can enjoy a variety of foods without digestive discomfort and have a robust immune system.

Vishama Agni (Irregular Agni): Typically associated with Vata dosha, Vishama Agni causes irregular digestion, where one day you may experience strong appetite and good digestion, while another day brings indigestion, gas, and bloating. This type of Agni benefits from grounding, warm, and nourishing foods.

Tikshna Agni (Intense Agni): Common in Pitta types, Tikshna Agni is an overly strong digestive fire that leads to fast digestion, often causing frequent hunger, acidity, and sometimes loose stools. Cooling, calming, and mild foods are recommended to soothe Tikshna Agni.

Manda Agni (Slow Agni): Usually associated with Kapha dosha, Manda Agni is a slow digestive fire that leads to sluggish digestion, heaviness, and sometimes constipation. Light, spicy, and invigorating foods can help stimulate Manda Agni.

Practical Tips for Cultivating Agni and Enhancing Digestion

Ayurveda offers practical ways to strengthen Agni, the digestive fire, essential for optimising digestion and reducing Ama, the residue of undigested food. Aligning diet, spices, and lifestyle with individual dosha needs supports a balanced digestive system and overall health. Eating meals at regular times and consuming freshly prepared, warm foods helps maintain Agni's strength. Spices like ginger, cumin, and fennel enhance digestion, transforming the relationship with food and well-being.

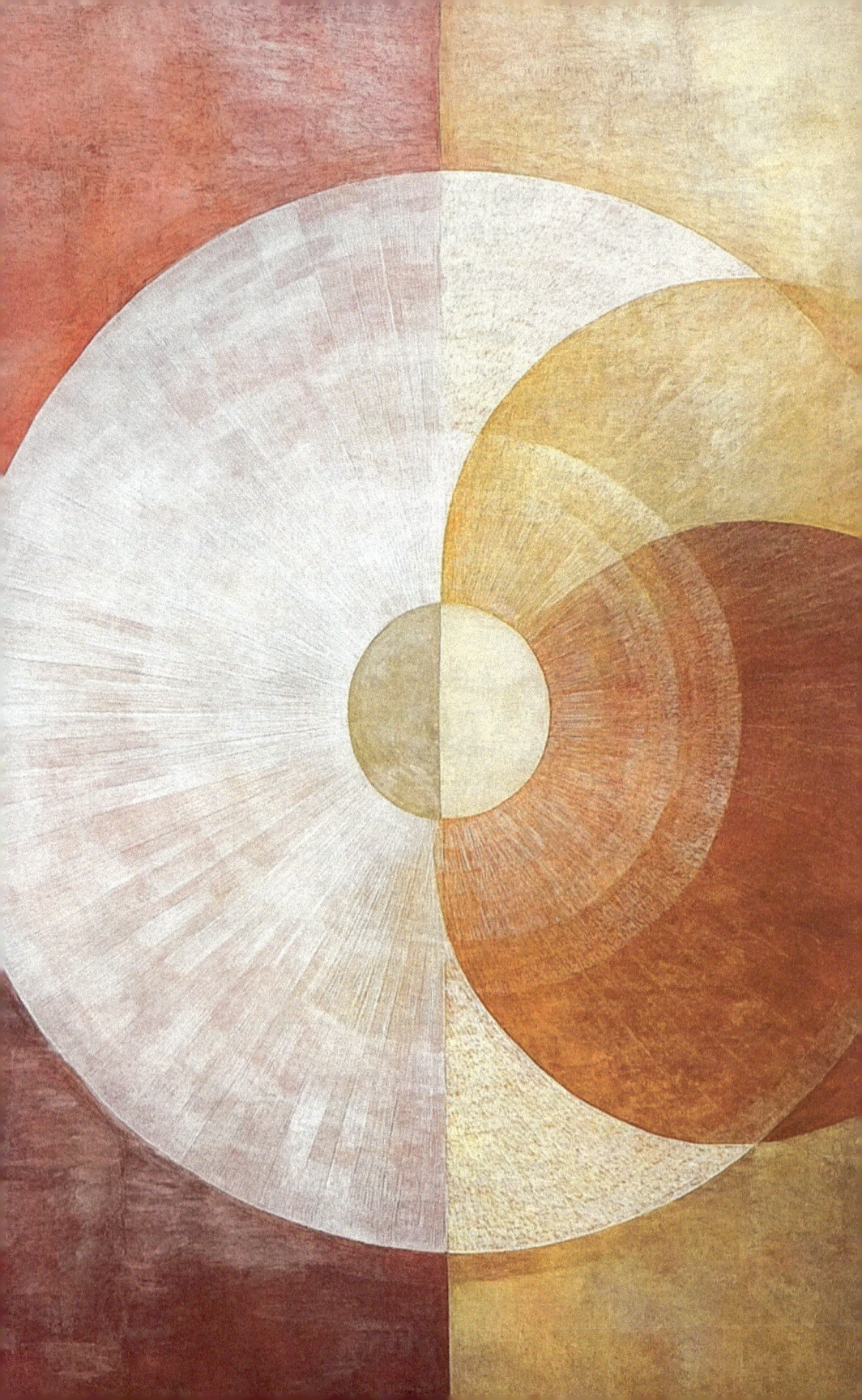

Guidelines For Each Dosha To Maintain Balanced Digestion:

Eating Mindfully

- Chew food thoroughly and avoid distractions while eating.
- Eat in a calm, pleasant environment, ideally without screens or rushed conversations.
- Practise gratitude before meals, setting an intention to nourish the body and mind.

Timing of Meals

- Eat Your Largest Meal at Midday: Agni is naturally strongest when the sun is highest, between 10 a.m. and 2 p.m., making midday the ideal time for the heaviest meal.
- Avoid Late Night Eating: Eating late in the evening can overwhelm digestion and lead to sluggishness and Ama accumulation.

Dosha-Specific Eating Habits

For Vata

- Focus on warm, cooked foods with healthy fats like ghee and olive oil to provide moisture and grounding.
- Include spices like ginger, cumin, and cinnamon to kindle Agni without overstimulation.
- Avoid cold, raw foods, which can be difficult for Vata to digest, especially in colder months.
- Eat at regular intervals, ideally three balanced meals, to reduce Vata's natural tendency toward erratic digestion.
- Include sweet, sour, and salty tastes in meals to balance Vata and encourage a sense of stability.
- Sip warm teas like chamomile or fennel throughout the day.
- Incorporate root vegetables like carrots and sweet potatoes.

31

For Pitta

- Emphasise cooling, hydrating foods like cucumber, leafy greens, fresh fruit, and coconut water to pacify Pitta's fiery Agni.
- Avoid excessively spicy, salty, or acidic foods, which can overstimulate digestion and increase internal heat.
- Focus on a balanced, moderate diet that includes cooling herbs like mint, coriander, and fennel.
- Include protein sources like legumes, beans, and moderate dairy, as Pitta has a strong appetite and often needs satisfying meals to maintain energy levels.

For Kapha

- Opt for lighter, spiced foods that stimulate digestion and reduce Kapha's sluggishness, such as ginger, black pepper, and turmeric.
- Minimise heavy, oily foods and refined sugars, which can contribute to Ama accumulation.
- Favour warm, cooked foods and limit dairy, cold foods, and overly sweet tastes, as these can dampen Agni.
- Practise portion control, as Kapha digestion is naturally slower, and lighter meals are often better tolerated.

Enhancing Digestion with Simple Ayurvedic Practices

Ayurveda offers various tools to enhance digestion and promote balanced Agni. Here are some simple yet effective practices to incorporate into your routine:

- **Drink Warm Water & Lemon in the Morning:** Starting the day with warm water and a squeeze of lemon can awaken Agni, flush out toxins, and prepare the digestive system for the day.
- **Use Digestive Spices:** Incorporating spices like cumin, fennel, ginger, and coriander into your meals can stimulate digestion, support metabolism, and prevent bloating.

- **Sip Warm Water or Herbal Tea with Meals:** Rather than drinking cold water, which can weaken Agni, sip warm water or herbal teas like ginger or fennel tea with meals to support digestion.
- **Avoid Overeating:** Ayurveda teaches that the stomach should be filled half with solid food, one-quarter with liquid, and left one-quarter empty to allow room for digestion. Overeating burdens Agni and leads to Ama.
- **Take a Short Walk After Eating:** A gentle walk after meals stimulates Agni and supports efficient digestion. Ayurveda suggests a light stroll rather than vigorous activity after meals to aid digestion without overwhelming it.

The Role of Ama in Health and Beauty

When Agni is weak, food is not completely digested, and the residue turns into a toxic substance called Ama. Ama accumulates in the digestive tract and eventually spreads throughout the body, obstructing energy flow, dulling the skin, and creating imbalances. Recognising and reducing Ama is essential for overall health and beauty.

Signs of Ama include:

- Coating on the tongue, particularly in the morning
- Sluggishness and lack of energy
- Brain fog and poor concentration
- Skin issues like breakouts or lacklustre complexion
- Digestive issues, such as gas, bloating, or irregular bowel movements

Ayurveda recommends regular cleansing practices, such as a simple detox routine, to help clear Ama. For example, incorporating a mono-diet of kitchari (a rice and lentil dish) for a day or two can give the digestive system a rest, allowing it to detoxify and reset. Pairing this with warm herbal teas, like ginger or coriander, can further support the cleansing process and enhance digestive fire.

Chapter 4

INTERNAL CLEANSING

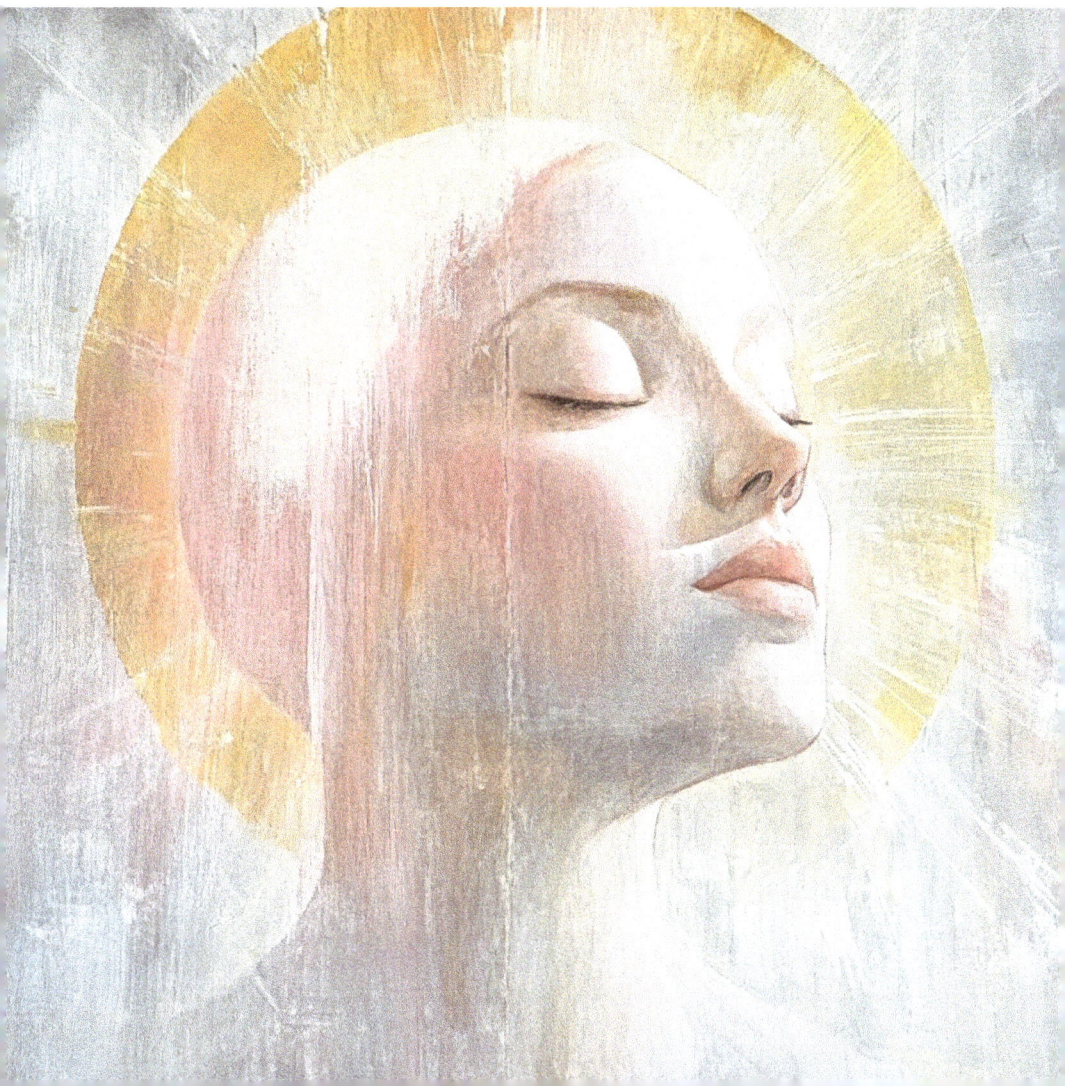

Inner Balance, The Secret Key,
For Glowing Skin And Vitality.
Gentle Cleansing, Toxins Release,
Restoring Beauty, Mind At Peace.

Chapter 4:
Drinking the Nectar
The Hydration Ritual

Ayurveda teaches that true beauty and health are reflections of inner purity and balance. When the body is free from toxins, the skin glows, energy levels are high, and the mind feels clear. Internal cleansing is not about extreme detoxes or harsh restrictions but rather a series of gentle, supportive practices that remove accumulated toxins and restore harmony in the body. This chapter introduces powerful Ayurvedic cleansing rituals that align with nature and can be easily integrated into daily routines.

Toxins, known as Ama in Ayurveda, accumulate due to incomplete digestion, unhealthy diet, stress, environmental pollutants, and other lifestyle factors. Over time, these toxins create blockages, hindering the flow of energy (prana) and affecting our overall well-being. Cleansing practices not only remove Ama but also rejuvenate the body, mind, and spirit, allowing our natural beauty to shine from within.

Secret 3: Inner Detox for Outer Radiance

The principle of "as within, so without" is central to Ayurvedic beauty. According to Ayurveda, our skin, hair, and overall appearance mirror the internal state of our health. Panchakarma, a cleansing system used in Ayurveda, is a powerful method for detoxifying the body and restoring balance. While some aspects of Panchakarma are performed by Ayurvedic practitioners, many cleansing techniques can be practiced at home.

Gentle Home Cleansing Practices

Tongue Scraping: Each morning, gently scrape your tongue using a stainless steel or copper tongue scraper. This removes the coating that forms overnight, a sign of toxins being eliminated through the digestive system. Tongue scraping freshens the breath and supports oral health. It's a simple yet powerful practice for better well-being.

Oil Pulling: Oil pulling involves swishing a tablespoon of oil (typically sesame or coconut) in the mouth for 10-15 minutes in the morning before eating. This practice helps draw out toxins from the mouth, strengthens gums, and can even improve oral health and skin clarity.

Triphala: Triphala is a traditional Ayurvedic herbal blend made from three fruits—Amalaki, Haritaki, and Bibhitaki. It gently supports digestion, elimination, and detoxification, promoting regular bowel movements and reducing Ama. Taken with warm water in the evening, Triphala supports natural detoxification.

Warm Water with Lemon: Drinking warm water with a squeeze of lemon first thing in the morning gently stimulates Agni and flushes toxins. This simple practice hydrates, kickstarts metabolism, and prepares the digestive system for the day.

Kitchari Cleanse: Kitchari, a nourishing dish made of rice and split mung beans, is easy to digest and a classic Ayurvedic cleansing meal. Eating kitchari for one or two days provides rest to the digestive system, allowing it to detoxify naturally and absorb nutrients more effectively.

Benefits of Regular Detoxification

By adopting these gentle cleansing practices, the body maintains balance, reduces Ama, and enhances energy flow. You may notice clearer skin, improved digestion, increased mental clarity, and a greater sense of vitality. The more we cleanse the body, the more it reflects on the outside, showing up as a vibrant, healthy appearance.

Secret 4: Drinking the Nectar – The Hydration Ritual

In Ayurveda, water is considered a source of life and energy. Proper hydration is essential for detoxification, nutrient transportation, and skin health. While hydration is important, Ayurveda emphasises the quality of water and how it's consumed, rather than simply increasing quantity.

Ayurvedic Hydration Tips

Warm Water with Lemon or Herbs: Starting the day with warm water and a squeeze of lemon, as mentioned, is not only a digestive stimulant but also a form of detox nectar. For additional benefits, consider adding herbs like ginger (for Vata), mint (for Pitta), or basil (for Kapha), to further balance your dosha and support digestion.

Sipping Warm Water Throughout the Day: Rather than gulping large amounts of cold water, Ayurveda suggests sipping warm water or herbal tea throughout the day. Cold water can weaken Agni, while warm water supports digestion, enhances circulation, and aids in flushing toxins.

Herbal Teas: Herbal teas are a nourishing way to stay hydrated while enhancing cleansing. Fennel, ginger, and cumin tea are particularly beneficial for digestion, while tulsi (holy basil) tea provides immune support and mental clarity. Choose teas that align with your dosha:

- **Vata:** Ginger, fennel, and liquorice tea to ground and warm.
- **Pitta:** Mint, hibiscus, and coriander tea to cool and soothe.
- **Kapha:** Ginger, cinnamon, and clove tea to invigorate and stimulate.

Coconut Water: For Pitta types or during hot weather, coconut water is a natural nectar with cooling and hydrating properties. It helps replenish electrolytes and refreshes the body without adding heat. Rich in essential minerals, it also supports healthy skin, boosts digestion, improves energy levels, and aids in calming an overactive mind.

Golden Milk: Golden milk, made with turmeric, warm milk (or plant-based milk), and a pinch of black pepper, is a nourishing bedtime drink. Turmeric is known for its anti-inflammatory and detoxifying properties, promoting a restful sleep and gentle cleansing during the night. A dash of cinnamon can enhance flavour, provide warmth, and offer additional nourishing and calming benefits.

Benefits of Ayurvedic Hydration Practices

Consuming water in a mindful, Ayurvedic way enhances the body's ability to detoxify, improves skin health, supports mental clarity, and maintains cellular vitality. By keeping the body hydrated with warm, herbal-infused water, you help flush out toxins and promote a natural glow, keeping both body and mind balanced and refreshed.

Secret 5: Body Exfoliation – Rejuvenating the Skin's Surface

Exfoliation is essential in Ayurveda for maintaining smooth, healthy, and vibrant skin. Regular body exfoliation removes dead skin cells, stimulates circulation, and supports the lymphatic system, which plays a crucial role in eliminating waste and toxins from the body.

Ayurvedic Body Exfoliation Techniques

Dry Brushing: Dry brushing involves using a natural-bristle brush to gently exfoliate the skin before bathing. Brush in long strokes toward the heart, starting from the feet and moving upward. Dry brushing stimulates the lymphatic system, improves circulation, and invigorates the skin.

Ubtan (Herbal Scrub): Ubtan is an Ayurvedic herbal paste made from natural ingredients such as chickpea flour, turmeric, sandalwood powder, and milk or rose water. It acts as a natural exfoliant and is especially effective in removing impurities from the skin, leaving it soft and glowing. Ubtan is gentle enough to use on the face and body.

Sugar Scrubs for Vata and Pitta: Sugar is gentler than salt and well-suited for dry Vata skin or sensitive Pitta skin. A sugar scrub made with sesame or coconut oil and a few drops of lavender or rose essential oil exfoliates gently while providing hydration and calming benefits. For an added touch of indulgence, mix in a teaspoon of honey to enhance moisturisation and leave your skin feeling silky smooth. Use this scrub in slow, circular motions to improve circulation to promote a healthy glow.

Salt Scrubs for Kapha: For Kapha types who may experience oily skin and water retention, a sea salt scrub infused with invigorating essential oils like eucalyptus or rosemary can effectively exfoliate and detoxify. Salt scrubs help draw out excess moisture and stimulate sluggish circulation, refreshing and toning the skin.

Benefits of Regular Exfoliation

Body exfoliation removes dull skin cells, enhances circulation, and promotes a natural glow. It also supports detoxification through the skin, which is the body's largest organ. Exfoliating regularly helps maintain a fresh, youthful appearance and provides a smooth canvas for oil treatments, allowing nourishing oils to penetrate deeper.

Secret 6: Oil Treatment – Nourishing the Body and Spirit

One of the most revered Ayurvedic beauty rituals is Abhyanga, or oil massage. Abhyanga involves massaging warm oil into the skin, which not only nourishes the skin but also relaxes the mind, soothes the nervous system, and supports overall wellness. This practice aligns with the Ayurvedic principle of "Snehana," or oleation, which literally means "to love or nurture." By anointing the body with oil, we foster a deep sense of self-care and self-love.

Dosha-Specific Oils and Techniques

- **Vata Balancing Oils:** Vata types benefit from warm, heavy, and grounding oils that counteract their naturally dry and light qualities. Sesame oil is ideal for Vata as it provides warmth and deep nourishment. Vata types can add a few drops of calming essential oils like lavender, vetiver, or geranium to enhance relaxation.
- **Pitta Balancing Oils:** Pitta types need cooling, soothing oils that reduce inflammation and calm their fiery energy. Coconut oil is naturally cooling and ideal for Pitta,

especially in warmer weather. Pitta types can enhance their oil massage with essential oils like sandalwood, rose, or chamomile for a calming effect.

- **Kapha Balancing Oils:** Kapha types benefit from warm, light, and stimulating oils that invigorate circulation and reduce heaviness. Mustard oil or almond oil infused with stimulating essential oils like eucalyptus, rosemary, or clary sage can provide warmth and enhance circulation, keeping Kapha balanced and energised.

Steps for a Traditional Abhyanga (Self-Oil Massage)

Warm the Oil: Pour your chosen oil into a small bowl and warm it gently by placing the bowl in a container of hot water. Warm oil is easier for the body to absorb and has a deeply relaxing effect on the nervous system.

Begin with the Head and Scalp: Apply a small amount of oil to the scalp and massage gently in circular motions. Oil massaging the scalp promotes relaxation, improves hair health, and nourishes the nervous system.

Massage the Body: Apply the oil generously to the rest of the body, using long strokes on the limbs and circular motions on the joints. Massage toward the heart to support lymphatic flow and stimulate circulation.

Allow the Oil to Absorb: After massaging the oil onto your skin, allow it to sit for 15–20 minutes before stepping into the shower. This resting period gives the oil time to penetrate deeply, nourishing and softening your skin from within. For an enhanced experience, use this time to relax, practise deep breathing, or engage in a short meditation to calm your mind and body, aligning your self-care routine with inner tranquillity.

Shower with Warm Water: Rinse off the oil using warm water to help open your pores and release impurities. Avoid using soap during this process, as the oil itself acts as a natural cleanser, leaving your skin moisturised, and glowing without stripping away its natural hydration.

Benefits of Oil Treatments

Abhyanga supports detoxification, calms the mind, and improves skin texture. The ritual also helps balance the nervous system, particularly or Vata types, who are prone to stress and anxiety. Practising Abhyanga regularly cultivates a radiant glow, leaving the skin deeply moisturised and creating a sense of inner calm and relaxation.

These cleansing rituals—inner detox, proper hydration, exfoliation, and oil treatment—are simple yet profound Ayurvedic practices that provide both internal and external benefits. Together, they form a powerful approach to beauty and wellness, grounding us in self-care and promoting a healthy, radiant glow that reflects inner harmony and vitality. Embracing these practices regularly fosters a sense of well-being, balance, and beauty that comes from deep within.

Chapter 5

SPIRITUAL HARMONY

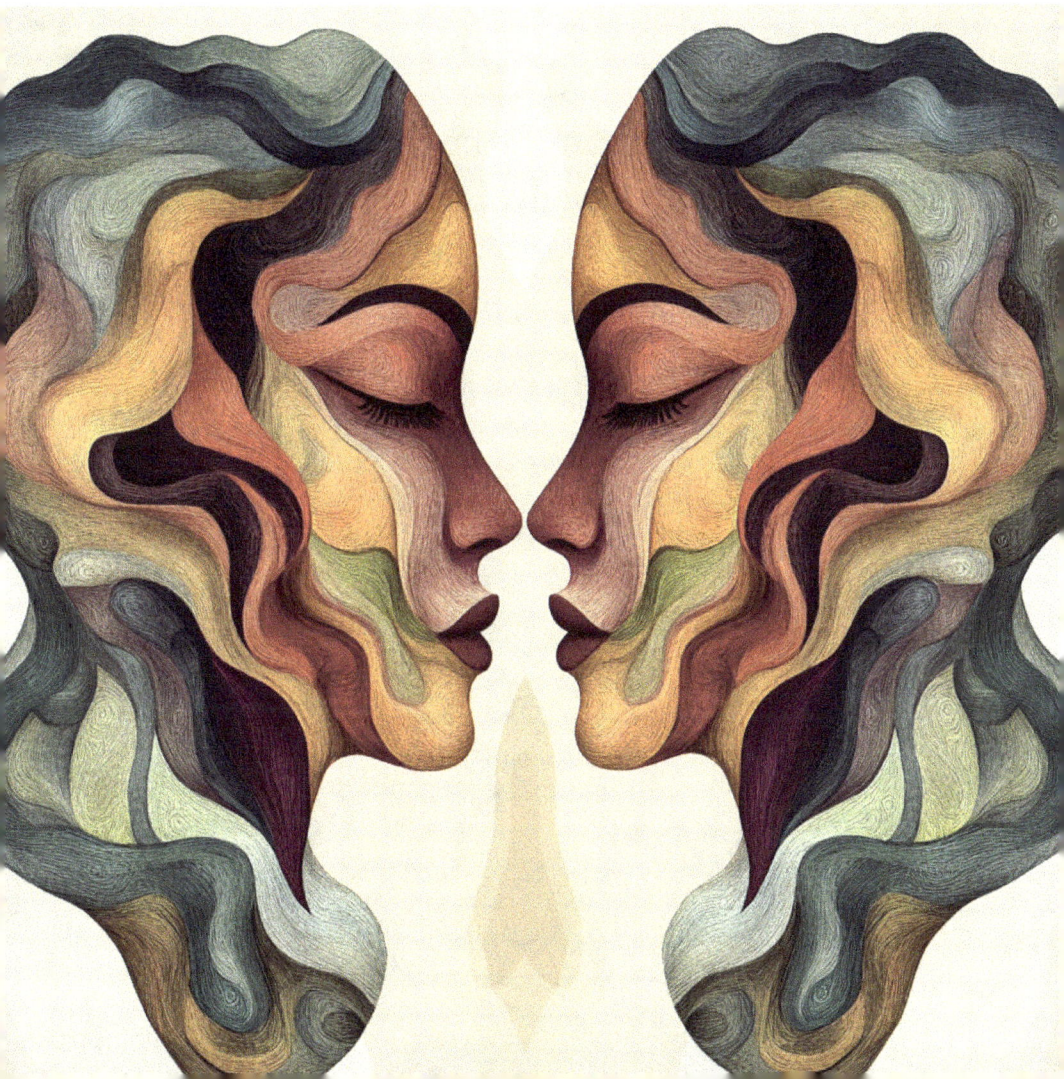

Radiance Blooms From Spirit Aligned,
A Balance Of Body, Heart, And Mind.
Through Subtle Layers, The Soul Takes Flight,
Ayurveda's Glow, Pure Inner Light.

Chapter 5:
Spiritual Harmony
Embracing Inner Peace

In Ayurveda, beauty is more than physical appearance; it is the radiance that emanates from a balanced and fulfilled spirit. True wellness encompasses not only the body but also the mind and soul. When we align with our deeper essence, we cultivate an inner glow that naturally expresses itself in our physical form. This chapter explores spiritual practices that connect us to our subtle energy bodies, helping us experience greater peace, resilience, and joy.

Ayurveda believes that each person is a microcosm of the universe, and that our health and happiness depend on our connection with the cosmic forces that shape our existence. This chapter introduces three secrets to achieving spiritual harmony: exploring the subtle bodies, practising pranayama, and finding joy in daily life. These practices help us move beyond physical beauty, fostering a radiance that comes from alignment with our highest self.

Secret 7: Exploring the Subtle Bodies – Understanding the Layers of Your Being

Ayurveda teaches that we are not merely physical bodies; we are composed of multiple layers, or subtle bodies, each of which plays a unique role in our well-being. Known as the Panchakosha or "five sheaths," these layers include the physical body, the energy body, the mental body, the wisdom body, and the bliss body. Together, they form a holistic view of human existence, encompassing both tangible and intangible aspects of our being.

Annamaya Kosha (Physical Body): This is the densest layer, representing the physical body, bones, muscles, and tissues. It is nourished by food and maintained through physical practices such as diet, exercise, mindful movement, and Ayurvedic routines. Caring for this layer supports overall vitality and well-being.

Pranamaya Kosha (Energy Body): This layer represents the flow of prana, or life force, within us. It encompasses the breath, circulatory system, and subtle energy pathways, or nadis. Pranamaya Kosha is balanced through pranayama, breathwork, and energy practices that enhance our vitality.

Manomaya Kosha (Mental Body): This layer is associated with the mind, emotions, and sensory perceptions. It is responsible for our thoughts, feelings, and reactions to the world around us. Practices such as meditation, mindfulness, and positive mental habits support the harmony of the mental body.

Vijnanamaya Kosha (Wisdom Body): Also known as the "intuitive" or "wisdom" body, this layer represents our ability to discern, reflect, and connect with higher knowledge. It is the seat of insight, self-awareness, and deeper understanding, accessed through introspection and spiritual study.

Anandamaya Kosha (Bliss Body): This is the innermost layer and is associated with a state of pure bliss and union with the universe. When we connect with this layer, we experience deep peace, joy, and spiritual fulfilment. It is accessed through deep meditation, self-realisation, and moments of spiritual alignment.

Balancing the Subtle Bodies

Each of the subtle bodies interacts with and influences the others. By nurturing all layers of our being, we achieve a state of holistic wellness that radiates outward. Here are ways to harmonise each layer:

Physical Body: Prioritise proper nutrition, physical activity, and sleep to maintain a strong foundation.

Energy Body: Practise pranayama and engage in mindful movement, such as yoga, to strengthen prana flow. Regular meditation can further harmonise and balance your energy.

Mental Body: Cultivate positive thoughts, engage in mindfulness, and avoid overstimulation to maintain mental clarity.

Wisdom Body: Engage in spiritual study, self-reflection, and practices that deepen understanding of life's purpose.

Bliss Body: Practise meditation, gratitude, and self-compassion to connect with the inner joy and peace.

Exploring the subtle bodies helps us understand our true nature, leading to a state of balance and harmony that enhances both inner and outer beauty.

Secret 8: Pranayama – Harnessing the Breath to Cultivate Inner Peace and Vitality

Pranayama, or the control of breath, is one of Ayurveda's most powerful tools for balancing the mind and body. Derived from the words "Prana" (life force) and "Ayama" (extension), pranayama refers to techniques that control and expand our life force through conscious breathing. Breath is the bridge between the body and the mind; by controlling it, we can influence our physical, mental, and emotional states.

Pranayama activates the Pranamaya Kosha (energy body) and clears the subtle energy channels (nadis), helping to release blockages that may hinder the free flow of prana. When prana flows freely, we experience greater mental clarity, emotional stability, and a sense of vitality. This practice also reduces stress and supports the nervous system, creating a calm and balanced state of mind that is essential for overall well-being.

Essential Pranayama Techniques

Nadi Shodhana (Alternate Nostril Breathing): This practice involves breathing through one nostril at a time, alternating in a controlled manner. Nadi Shodhana balances the left and right hemispheres of the brain, harmonises prana, and is especially beneficial for calming Vata and balancing the mind.

How to Practise:
Sit comfortably, close your right nostril with your thumb, inhale through the left nostril, close the left nostril with your ring finger, exhale through the right nostril, then inhale through the right, and exhale through the left. Repeat for 5-10 minutes.

Kapalabhati (Skull Shining Breath): This is an energising technique involving rapid, forceful exhalations followed by passive inhalations. Kapalabhati increases blood flow, boosts metabolism, and is ideal for clearing mental fog and energising Kapha.

How to Practise: Take a deep breath in, then exhale sharply through the nose, pulling in the belly with each exhale. Repeat in a rhythmic manner for 1-2 minutes.

Bhramari (Bee Breath): This technique involves humming during exhalation, creating a sound that soothes the mind and calms the nervous system. Bhramari is particularly helpful for Pitta, as it reduces internal heat and tension.

How to Practise: Close your eyes, take a deep breath in, and as you exhale, produce a gentle humming sound like a bee. Focus on the vibrations within your body. Repeat 5-7 times.

Shitali (Cooling Breath): Shitali involves breathing in through a rolled tongue, which cools the air and calms the body and mind. It is an effective practice for reducing excess heat and calming Pitta. This technique soothes the nervous system and promotes a sense of relaxation. Regular practice can help manage stress and enhance overall well-being.

How to Practise: Roll your tongue, inhale through the mouth, close your mouth, and exhale through the nose. Repeat for 5-10 breaths.

Benefits of Pranayama

Pranayama harmonises the body's energy, reduces stress, and promotes mental clarity. When practised regularly, it can boost immunity, support emotional resilience, and improve overall vitality. By bringing attention to the breath, pranayama connects us with the present moment, allowing us to cultivate a profound sense of inner peace and a radiant energy that reflects outward.

Secret 9: Find Your Joy – Embracing the Path to Inner Fulfilment

Ayurveda teaches that joy is the natural state of the soul. When we are aligned with our true nature, joy flows effortlessly, and this inner happiness shines through, enhancing our vitality, appearance, and well-being. However, the demands of modern life often pull us away from this inner joy, leading to stress, dissatisfaction, and imbalance. Finding joy is not about seeking pleasure externally but about reconnecting with the deeper wellspring of fulfilment within.

Joy in Ayurveda is connected to the Anandamaya Kosha, or bliss body, which is the deepest layer of our being. When we are aligned with this layer, we experience a sense of completeness, contentment, and connection to the universe. Practising gratitude, engaging in activities we love, and spending time in nature are all ways to access this inner joy and cultivate a more radiant life.

Practices to Cultivate Joy

Gratitude Meditation: Practising gratitude helps us focus on the positive aspects of our lives and creates a sense of abundance and appreciation. Each day, spend a few minutes reflecting on things you are grateful for. This shifts your focus away from stress and towards a feeling of contentment.

Pursuing Creative Outlets: Creativity is an expression of the soul. Engaging in creative activities—whether it's painting, writing, dancing, or gardening—allows us to express ourselves fully and connect with our inner joy. Ayurveda encourages making time for hobbies and activities that nourish our spirit.

Connecting with Nature: Spending time in nature reminds us of our connection to the larger universe and restores a sense of balance. Whether it's a walk in the park, a hike in the mountains, or simply sitting under a tree, connecting with nature brings peace and joy to the soul.

Practising Kindness and Compassion: Ayurveda views kindness as a healing force. Performing acts of kindness—whether for others or yourself—promotes feelings of warmth, connection, and joy. Practise compassion for yourself and others, and notice how it lifts your spirit.

Chapter 6

ESSENTIAL OILS

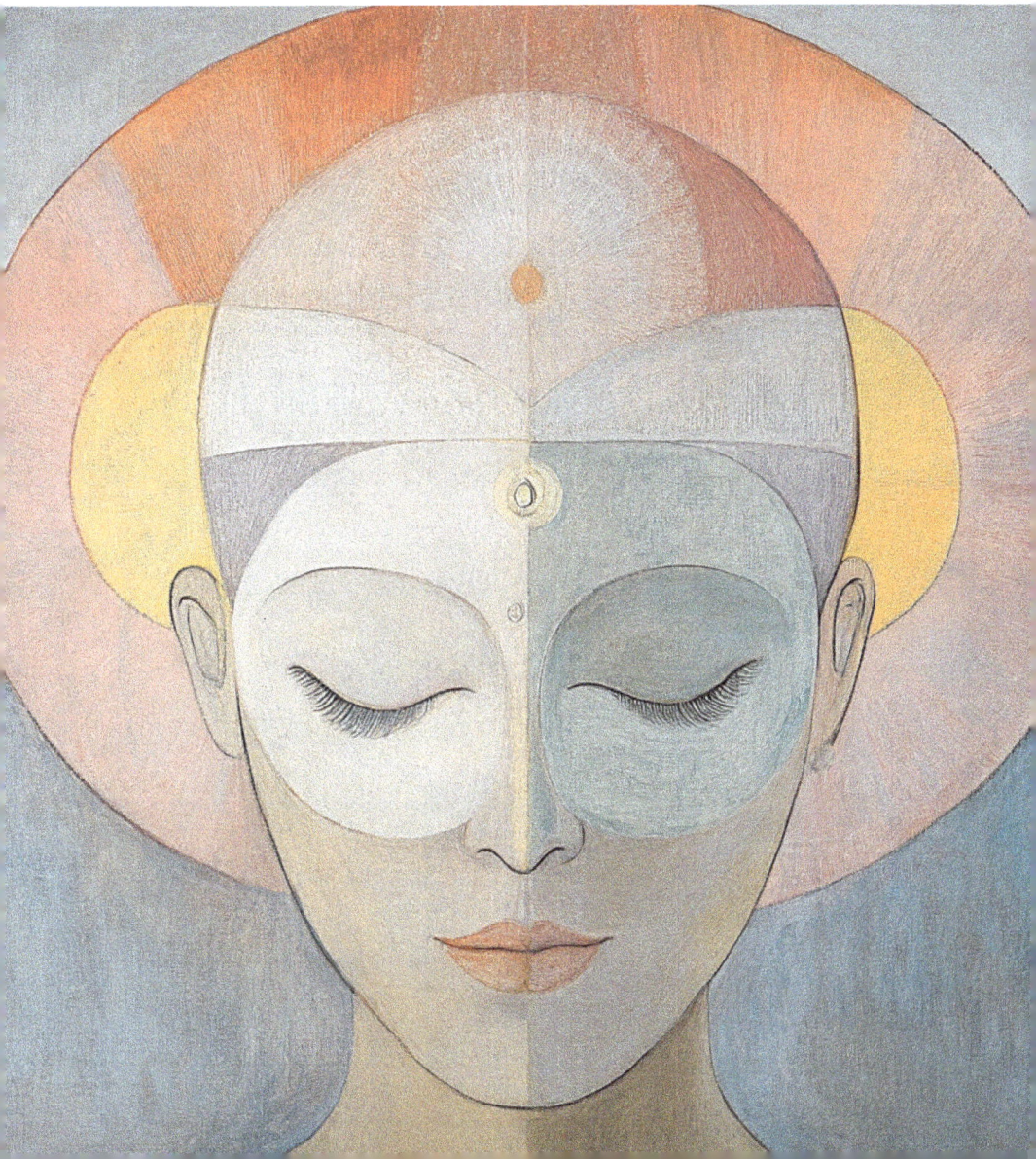

Nature's Essence, Pure And True,
Nurtures Skin With Healing Hue.
Dosha-Aligned, They Bring To Light,
Harmony's Glow, Soft And Bright.

Chapter 6:
Essential Oils
Harnessing Nature's Essence

Essential oils have been used for thousands of years in Ayurveda for their therapeutic, balancing, and beautifying properties. These concentrated plant essences contain powerful nutrients, antioxidants, and healing compounds that promote physical and emotional well-being. Ayurveda embraces essential oils as part of a holistic approach to skincare, integrating them into daily routines to nurture the skin, balance the mind, and create a sense of harmony.

In Ayurvedic beauty, essential oils are carefully selected to align with an individual's dosha and skin type. Because each dosha has unique characteristics and needs, essential oils offer a tailored approach, allowing you to address specific skin concerns while bringing balance to your constitution. Whether you need hydration, calming effects, or gentle exfoliation, the right essential oils can become potent allies in your journey to radiant skin.

This chapter explores how to use essential oils for your dosha, combining them with carrier oils, and integrating them into a balanced skincare routine. Secret 10, "The Right Skincare for You," offers detailed insights into choosing oils and products that best support your Ayurvedic beauty goals.

Secret 10: The Right Skincare For You – Customising Ayurvedic Beauty With Essential Oils

Selecting skincare begins with understanding your dosha and its influence on your skin type. In Ayurveda, skincare honours individual uniqueness rather than adopting a one-size-fits-all approach. Essential oils offer a personalised method to address specific skin needs according to doshic imbalances. The following sections guide you in choosing essential oils for Vata, Pitta, and Kapha skin types.

Vata Skin: Nourishment and Hydration

Vata skin, governed by the elements of Air and Ether, tends to be dry, delicate, and prone to premature ageing. Vata skin is typically thin, with a tendency toward roughness and fine lines, especially in colder or drier climates. Vata skin benefits from oils that provide deep nourishment, hydration, and protection against environmental stressors.

Essential Oils for Vata:

Rose: Rose oil is deeply hydrating, soothing, and rejuvenating for dry skin. Its gentle aroma also calms the mind and reduces Vata-induced anxiety.

Sandalwood: Sandalwood has natural emollient properties, helping to lock in moisture while balancing dry, rough skin. It is cooling and grounding, perfect for stabilising Vata.

Frankincense: Known for its anti-ageing properties, frankincense supports cell regeneration, reduces fine lines, and enhances elasticity.

Geranium: Geranium oil balances moisture levels and is excellent for sensitive or flaky skin, helping to soothe dryness and inflammation.

Carrier Oils for Vata:

Sesame Oil: Rich, warming, and deeply hydrating, sesame oil is ideal for Vata skin. It helps to restore moisture, reduce roughness, and protect the skin from the elements. Additionally, sesame oil's antioxidant properties support skin health and combat signs of ageing. Regular application can enhance skin elasticity and promote a radiant complexion.

Almond Oil: Lightweight and nourishing, almond oil absorbs easily, hydrating and softening Vata skin with essential fatty acids. Rich in vitamin E, it repairs damage, improves texture, soothes inflammation, and alleviates dryness and irritation linked to Vata imbalances.

Skincare Ritual for Vata:

Daily Cleanse: Use a gentle, creamy cleanser with a few drops of rose or sandalwood oil to hydrate and soothe the skin.

Moisturise with Warm Oil: Apply a blend of sesame or almond oil infused with frankincense or geranium after cleansing. Warm the oil slightly before applying to enhance absorption.

Weekly Mask: Create a nourishing mask with honey, aloe vera, and a drop of geranium oil for added hydration and a radiant glow.

Pitta Skin: Cooling and Calming

Pitta skin, governed by Fire and Water, is typically sensitive, prone to inflammation, and may exhibit redness, rashes, or acne. Pitta skin is often medium in thickness with a warm undertone. The goal for Pitta skincare is to soothe, cool, and protect the skin from excess heat, helping to prevent breakouts and calm inflammation.

Essential Oils for Pitta:

Lavender: Lavender oil is cooling, calming, and anti-inflammatory, making it ideal for reducing redness and soothing sensitive skin.

Chamomile: Chamomile has gentle anti-inflammatory and healing properties, helping to calm irritation and reduce Pitta-related sensitivity. Its soothing nature promotes balance and relaxation.

Rose: Cooling and balancing, rose oil soothes Pitta's fiery nature, reduces redness, and keeps the skin hydrated.

Ylang Ylang: This essential oil balances oil production and has a calming effect on the mind, making it beneficial for Pitta types prone to stress-induced breakouts.

Carrier Oils for Pitta:

Coconut Oil: Coconut oil's cooling nature is ideal for Pitta skin. It hydrates, soothes, and reduces redness, making it perfect for sensitive or acne-prone skin.

Sunflower Oil: Sunflower oil is light, non-comedogenic, and hydrating, with cooling properties that help calm Pitta skin.
Skincare Ritual for Pitta:

Daily Cleanse: Use a gentle gel or cream cleanser with a few drops of lavender or chamomile oil to remove impurities and calm the skin.

Moisturise with Cooling Oil: Apply coconut or sunflower oil with added rose or ylang ylang oil to keep skin moisturised and reduce redness.

Weekly Mask: Mix cooling ingredients like cucumber, aloe vera, and a drop of chamomile or lavender oil into a mask to soothe inflammation and cool the skin.

Kapha Skin: Stimulation and Detoxification

Kapha skin, governed by Earth and Water, is usually thick, oily, and resilient. While Kapha skin is less prone to wrinkles and ageing, it often suffers from excess oil, enlarged pores, and a tendency toward congestion and acne. Kapha skin benefits from oils that are light, stimulating, and purifying to balance oil production and maintain clarity.

Essential Oils for Kapha:

Tea Tree: Tea tree oil is antibacterial, purifying, and effective for controlling excess oil and breakouts.

Eucalyptus: Eucalyptus oil is invigorating and helps to decongest the skin, promoting clarity and balance.

Rosemary: Rosemary oil has astringent properties that tighten the skin and reduce excess oil, making it ideal for Kapha.

Grapefruit: Grapefruit oil is refreshing, detoxifying, and promotes a radiant complexion by reducing Kapha's excess oil.
Carrier Oils for Kapha:

Grapeseed Oil: Light and astringent, grapeseed oil absorbs quickly without clogging pores, helping to control oil production.

Jojoba Oil: Jojoba oil balances oil production and mimics the skin's natural oils, making it a great choice for Kapha skin.
Skincare Ritual for Kapha:

Daily Cleanse: Use a gel or foaming cleanser with a drop of tea tree or eucalyptus oil to purify and prevent congestion.

Light Moisturising: Use grapeseed or jojoba oil with a drop of rosemary or grapefruit oil for hydration without heaviness.

Weekly Exfoliation: Kapha skin benefits from regular exfoliation. Use an ubtan (Ayurvedic scrub) made from chickpea flour, turmeric, and a drop of tea tree oil to remove dead skin cells, reduce oil, and improve texture.

Creating Your Ayurvedic Skincare Routine with Essential Oils

Each dosha-specific skincare ritual can be further customised based on your environment, season, and current skin condition. Essential oils can be added to cleansers, masks, and moisturisers or applied directly to the skin (diluted in a carrier oil) for targeted benefits. Here's how to incorporate them into a simple Ayurvedic skincare routine:

Cleansing: Begin by cleansing the skin with a dosha-appropriate cleanser infused with essential oils. Vata types may prefer a creamy cleanser with rose oil, Pitta types a gel with chamomile, and Kapha types a foaming cleanser with tea tree or eucalyptus.

Toning: Create a simple toner by adding 1-2 drops of essential oil to distilled water. Rose water or witch hazel with lavender or sandalwood works well for Pitta and Vata, while Kapha can benefit from witch hazel with rosemary.

Moisturising: After cleansing and toning, apply a blend of carrier and essential oils suited to your skin type. Lightly warm the oil in your hands before pressing it gently onto the face to encourage absorption.

Weekly Treatments: Use masks, exfoliants, and oils for deeper treatments once or twice a week. Essential oils can be added to natural masks, scrubs, and exfoliants based on your skin's current needs.

Self-Massage: Incorporate a gentle self-massage using your chosen oils to stimulate circulation, relax the facial muscles, and improve lymphatic drainage. This not only enhances the skin's radiance but also promotes a calm and centred mind.

Conclusion

EMBRACING AYURVEDA

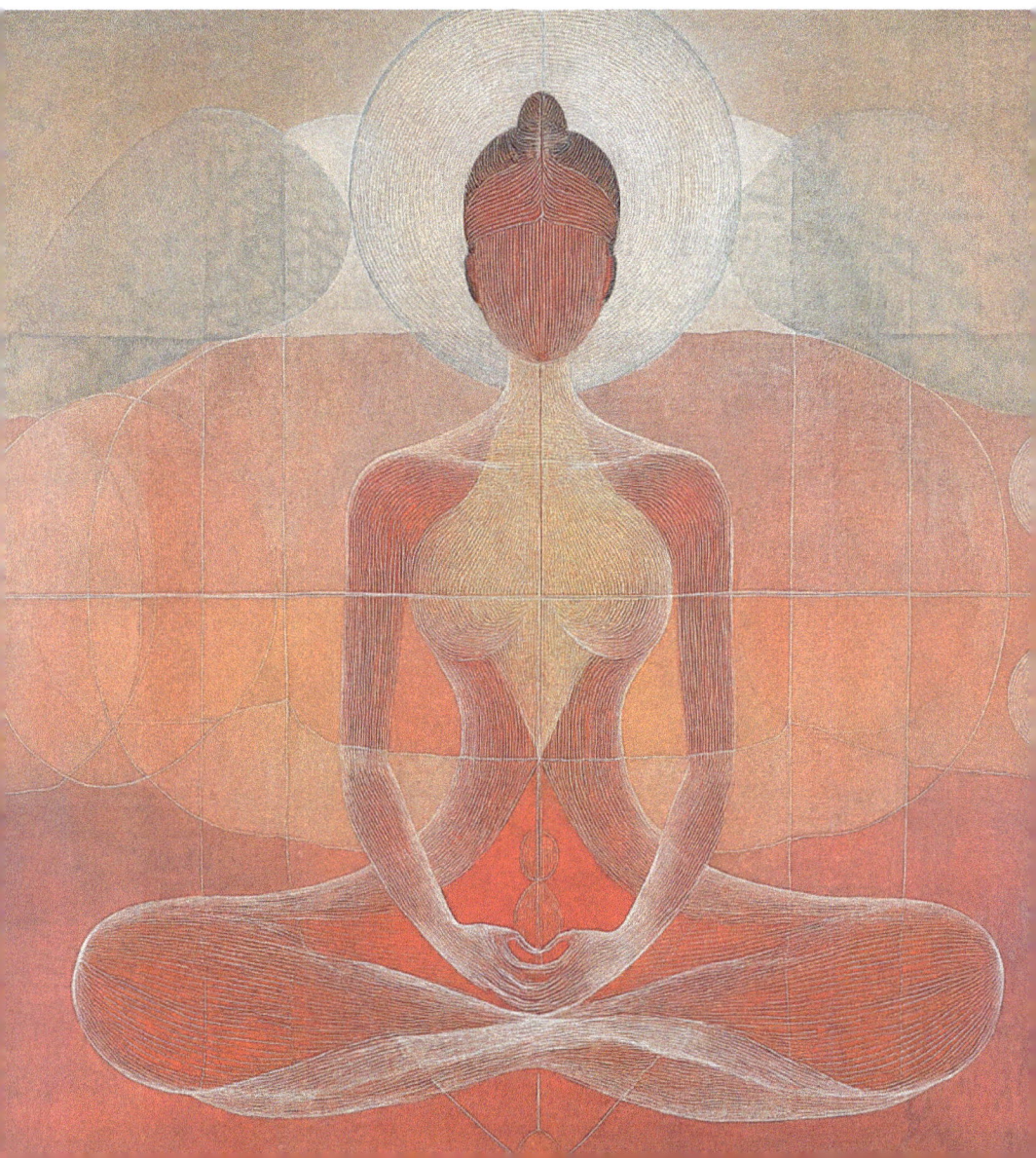

True Beauty Flows From A Peaceful Heart,
A Timeless Glow, Where Balance Starts.
Ayurveda Guides With Wisdom's Grace,
To Nurture The Soul And Light The Face

Conclusion
Embracing Ayurveda
As a Life Long Journey

As you reach the end of this journey through Ayurvedic beauty, I hope you feel empowered with a deeper understanding of how true beauty stems from inner harmony. Ayurveda teaches us that beauty is more than a fleeting appearance; it is the radiance that emerges when we live in balance, align with our unique nature, and nurture our body, mind, and spirit. This ancient science provides us with holistic practices that go beyond skincare, inviting us to care for ourselves on every level.

Through Ayurveda, you've discovered that beauty is not something to be pursued or achieved; it is something that reveals itself when we honour and nourish our true selves. Each of the ten secrets you've explored—from understanding your dosha to cultivating Agni, practising mindful cleansing, and nurturing your inner joy—contributes to a deeper transformation, one that extends far beyond the surface.

The Power of Gentle Shifts

Remember, Ayurveda is a journey—a series of gentle shifts that bring us closer to our truest, most radiant selves. Small, consistent changes make the most lasting impact, whether it's starting each day with warm water and lemon, setting aside time for a self-oil massage, or incorporating essential oils that resonate with your dosha. The journey may start with simple practices, but these practices have the potential to transform how you feel, think, and experience life.

Ayurveda reminds us to embrace the ebb and flow of life, accepting that our needs will change with the seasons, our environment, and the experiences we encounter. This dynamic approach to self-care encourages us to listen to our bodies and adjust our routines accordingly. There will be days when your skin needs extra nourishment, when your mind craves stillness, or when your heart yearns for joy and connection. Allow Ayurveda to be a supportive framework that guides you in meeting these changing needs.

Beauty as a Reflection of Inner Harmony

The Ayurvedic journey is ultimately a path toward self-discovery. True beauty radiates from within when we are aligned with who we are and feel at peace with ourselves. As you move forward, may these principles empower you to honour your body as a temple, care for your mind as a source of wisdom, and nurture your spirit as the essence of your being.

As you apply these Ayurvedic practices, you'll find that beauty becomes a natural byproduct of living in harmony. Instead of striving for perfection, Ayurveda invites you to celebrate your unique beauty, embracing every line, curve, and feature as a testament to your journey. Let your radiant self be a reminder of your commitment to self-care, self-love, and balance.

Moving Forward: A Lifelong Commitment to Self-Care

The journey of Ayurveda is lifelong, and each step brings you closer to your natural state of well-being. As you incorporate these practices into your daily life, you are investing in the most precious gift—your own health, vitality, and happiness. Ayurvedic beauty isn't a quick fix; it's a commitment to yourself, a promise to nurture your inner light and allow it to shine brightly in the world.

Let these teachings inspire you as you navigate life's challenges, reminding you that peace and beauty reside within. Whether you're just beginning your Ayurvedic journey or deepening your practice, every choice to balance, nourish, and love yourself is a step toward a more fulfilling and radiant life. Thank you for allowing Ayurveda to become part of your journey. May your path be filled with harmony, joy, and endless discovery as you unlock the secrets of beauty within.

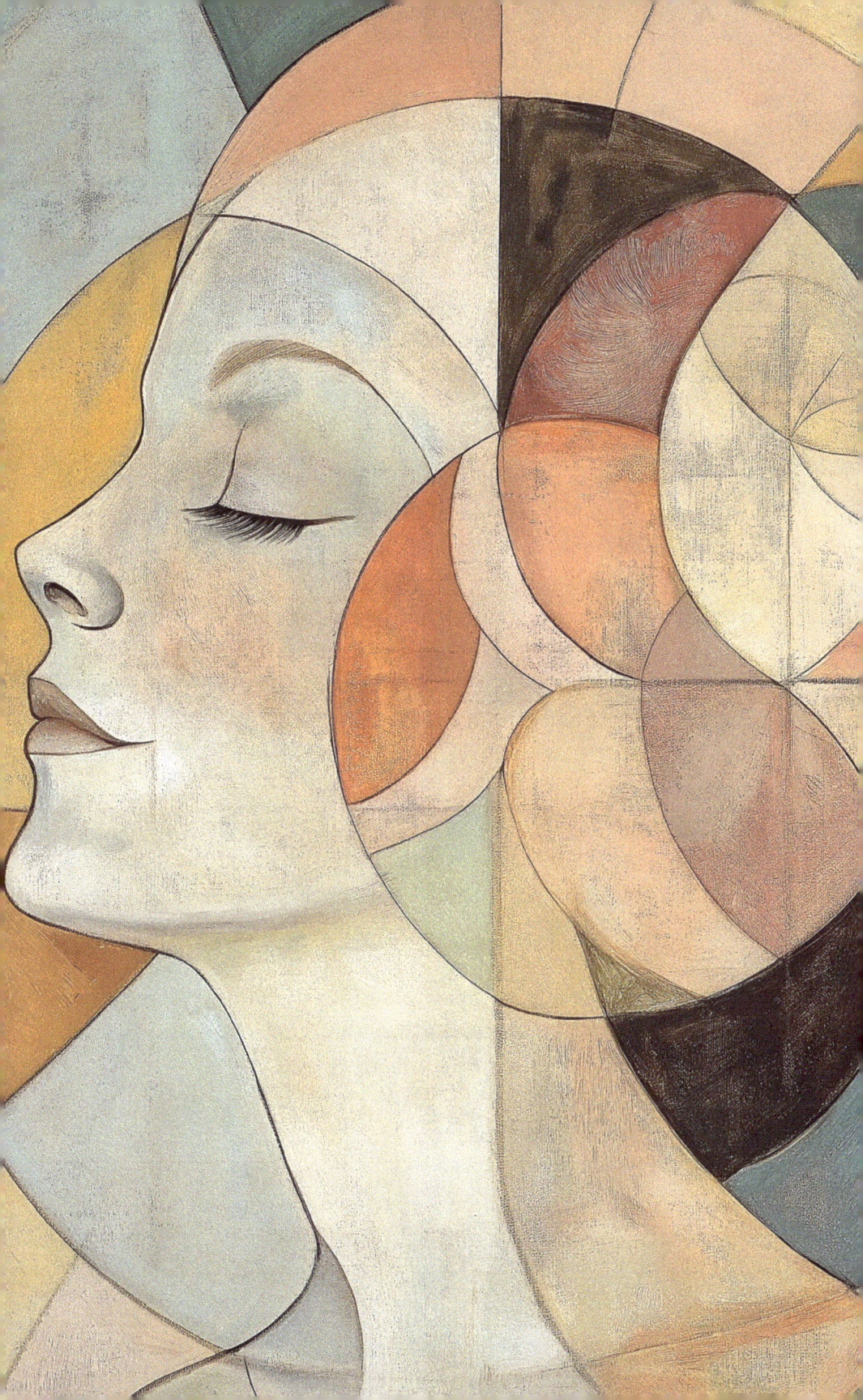

Glossary of Ayurvedic Terms

Agni (ahg-nee)
The Sanskrit word for "fire," Agni represents the digestive fire in Ayurveda. It governs digestion, absorption, and assimilation of food and experiences. A balanced Agni is essential for vitality and wellness, while an imbalanced Agni leads to toxins (Ama).

Ama (ah-mah)
Ama refers to toxins or undigested residues that accumulate in the body due to weak Agni. It is considered the root cause of many health issues, including sluggishness, dull skin, and digestive problems.

Anandamaya Kosha (ah-nahn-dah-my-yah koh-shah)
The "bliss body," this is the innermost of the five sheaths (Panchakosha). It represents pure joy and spiritual fulfilment, accessible through deep meditation and alignment with one's true nature.

Annamaya Kosha (ahn-nah-my-yah koh-shah)
The "physical body" or the outermost layer of the Panchakosha, representing the tangible aspects of the body such as muscles, bones, and tissues. It is nourished by proper diet and exercise.

Abhyanga (uhb-yuhn-gah)
A traditional Ayurvedic self-massage using warm oils tailored to an individual's dosha. Abhyanga nourishes the skin, soothes the nervous system, and promotes relaxation and detoxification.

Dinacharya (dee-nah-char-yah)
Ayurvedic daily routine, designed to promote health and balance. It includes practices such as oil pulling, tongue scraping, meditation, and eating meals at regular times.

Dosha (doh-shah)

The three primary energies or bio-elements—Vata, Pitta, and Kapha—that govern all physical, mental, and emotional processes in the body. Each person has a unique combination of doshas that shapes their constitution (Prakruti).

- Vata: Composed of Air and Ether, it governs movement and creativity.
- Pitta: Made of Fire and Water, it governs digestion and transformation.
- Kapha: Comprised of Earth and Water, it governs structure and stability.

Kitchari (kit-cha-ree)

A simple, nourishing Ayurvedic dish made from rice and split mung beans. Often used in detoxes, it is easy to digest and supports cleansing and rejuvenation.

Manomaya Kosha (mah-noh-my-yah koh-shah)

The "mental body," representing the mind and emotions. This layer influences thoughts, feelings, and sensory perceptions. It is harmonised through mindfulness and meditation.

Nadi (nah-dee)

Subtle energy channels through which prana (life force) flows in the body. Blocked nadis can lead to imbalances, which can be corrected through practices like pranayama and yoga.

Panchakosha (pahn-chah-koh-shah)

The "five sheaths" or layers of human existence in Ayurveda. These include the physical body (Annamaya), energy body (Pranamaya), mental body (Manomaya), wisdom body (Vijnanamaya), and bliss body (Anandamaya).

Prakruti (prah-kroo-tee)

An individual's unique constitution, determined at birth, comprising a specific balance of the three doshas. It defines inherent tendencies and health predispositions.

Pranamaya Kosha (prah-nah-my-yah koh-shah)

The "energy body," which includes the breath and subtle life force (prana). Balanced through pranayama and energy work, it supports vitality and well-being.

Prana (prah-nah)

The life force or vital energy that sustains all living beings. It flows through the body via nadis and is regulated by breath.

Pranayama (prah-nah-yah-mah)

Breath control practices in Ayurveda and yoga. Pranayama techniques, such as Nadi Shodhana and Bhramari, balance the mind, regulate energy, and promote inner peace.

Ritucharya (ree-too-char-yah)

Seasonal routines in Ayurveda that align diet, exercise, and lifestyle practices with the changing seasons to maintain balance and health throughout the year.

Snehana (sneh-hah-nah)

A term meaning "to love or nurture," often associated with oleation (oil treatments) in Ayurveda. It includes practices like Abhyanga, which deeply nourish and soothe the body.

Triphala (tri-phah-lah)

A traditional Ayurvedic herbal blend of three fruits—Amalaki, Haritaki, and Bibhitaki. It supports digestion, detoxification, and rejuvenation.

Ubtan (oob-tahn)
A traditional Ayurvedic herbal scrub made from natural ingredients like chickpea flour, turmeric, and sandalwood. Used for exfoliation, it promotes clear, glowing skin.

Vikruti (vik-roo-tee)
A temporary imbalance in the doshas caused by factors such as stress, poor diet, or seasonal changes. Ayurveda aims to restore Vikruti to the individual's natural state (Prakruti).

Vijnanamaya Kosha (vee-gyah-nah-my-yah koh-shah)
The "wisdom body," representing insight and higher knowledge. It is cultivated through introspection, self-reflection, and spiritual practices.

www.ingramcontent.com/pod-product-compliance
Lightning Source LLC
Chambersburg PA
CBHW072213270326
41930CB00011B/2621